Review of Neurology

A Workbook for Speech and Hearing Students

Review of Neurology

A Workbook for Speech and Hearing Students

Jayanti Ray, PhD, CCC-SLP

Department of Speech and Hearing Sciences
Washington State University
Pullman, Washington

With 70 Illustrations

M Mosby

An Affiliate of Elsevier

An Affiliate of Elsevier

11830 Westline Industrial Drive
St. Louis, Missouri 63146

REVIEW OF NEUROLOGY: A WORKBOOK FOR SPEECH AND HEARING STUDENTS   0-323-02297-9

Publishing Director: Linda Duncan
Acquisitions Editor: Kathy Falk
Developmental Editor: Jennifer Watrous
Publishing Services Manager: Deborah L. Vogel
Senior Project Manager: Ann E. Rogers
Senior Book Designer: Bill Drone

Printed in the United States of America.

Last digit is the print number: 9   8   7   6   5   4   3   2   1

Preface

"We sit on the threshold of important new advances in neuroscience that will yield increased understanding of how the brain functions and the more effective treatments to heal brain disorders and diseases. How the brain behaves in health and disease may well be the most important question in our lifetime."

Richard D. Broadwell, from Neuroscience, Memory, and the Brain, 1995

This workbook attempts to synthesize necessary neurological information for the purpose of immersing students of the speech and hearing sciences into the field of neurology. The objective is a deeper understanding of the complexities of the human nervous system and its disorders. This workbook presents practical information that should help speech and hearing students better understand neurological concepts.

Neurology is the study of the nervous system with an emphasis on its structures, functions, and abnormalities. The human nervous system is a highly complex and organized system, representing a dynamic network of neurons. Neuropathological conditions are the foundation for various speech, language, and cognition deficits, so it is important to develop concepts pertinent to neuroanatomy, neurophysiology, and neuropathology. In my teaching experience, I have found that students gain proper insight into neurological communication disorders only when they have had clinical experience and have looked at clinical examples using a problem-based learning approach. Thus I have incorporated various case studies to enhance students' clinical concepts.

The material presented in each chapter is designed to help refresh already learned concepts and allow easy retrieval of information. Each chapter is accompanied by a short text that covers the most important and basic information. This workbook is focused on reinforcing student learning and retention via various question-and-answer formats and case studies. The goal is to help students apply neurological concepts effectively in clinical situations.

The 15 chapters in this book present an overall conceptualization of the nervous system, starting with the neuron and moving through specific neuropathological conditions. Information is presented in the following five distinct formats: (1) clinical notes, (2) tables, (3) summaries, (4) question-and-answer sections, and (5) illustrations, specifically, schematic diagrams.

Chapter 1 provides a brief tour of the building blocks of the nervous system, dealing with neurons, neuronal physiology, and supporting cells. Chapter 2 offers a basic understanding of the complex architecture of the human nervous system. Chapter 3 deals with the major divisions of the brain and how the brain is responsible for various vital functions and behaviors. Chapter 4 covers the ventricular system and blood supply to the brain. The cranial nerves are described in Chapter 5. It is vital that speech and hearing students understand neuropathological conditions related to the cranial nerves because of the relationship between cranial nerve lesions and speech and swallowing functions. Cranial nerve disorders are systematically presented in the multiple-choice question format, which walks readers through the most common neuropathological conditions. Chapters 6, 7, and 8 present an outline of the sensory pathways that carry information about audition, vision, balance, and other sensations. Chapter 9 deals with the motor pathways that regulate various crude and skilled motor movements. Chapter 10 emphasizes the role of cortical and subcortical centers needed in processing speech and language. The main disorders of the cerebral cortex (including aphasia, apraxia, dementia, agnosia) are explained. An outline of the neurological examination is presented in Chapter 11, with most of the content related to neurodiagnostic tests covered in the question-and-answer section. The development of the nervous system across the life span is discussed in Chapters 12 and 13, along with various nervous system disorders that result from aging. Chapters 14 and 15 deal with problem-based learning, offering case studies in both pediatric and adult populations. Logically sequenced multiple-choice questions have been presented to help students understand complex neuroanatomical correlates, behaviors, and pathological factors in various neurological conditions.

Appendixes present important supplementary information for speech-language pathologists. The information offered includes nerve supplies to muscles important for swallowing and speech functions; assessment of adults with neurogenic communication disorders; neurological examinations to be used by the speech-language pathologist; and important websites with information on neuroanatomy and neurodiagnostics. Two detailed self-examinations for all of the chapters are also included. The bibliography offers a comprehensive list of references.

I hope students will find this comprehensive workbook useful in reviewing their understanding of neuroanatomy and neuropathological conditions related to communication disorders.

ACKNOWLEDGMENTS

This book is dedicated to the students who use it.

This workbook on neurology would not have been possible without the help of many individuals who have supported my ideas and helped me unconditionally to develop my work.

My heartfelt thanks to my husband, Nirmal, and to my sons, Jade and Justin, who have toiled hard along with me during the preparation of this book.

My gratitude to my guide, Dr. P.R. Terraiya; my parents; and my brother for their continuing inspiration.

Many thanks to my students in neurology classes, who have always taught me in the classroom and have made my work easier.

My sincere thanks to Jennifer Watrous, Kellie Fitzpatrick, and Ann Rogers of Elsevier, who always lent their helping hands whenever I needed.

My thanks to my mentor Dr. Jean Johnson for her encouragement and support.

And lastly, I thank Dr. Chermak, the chair of the Department of Speech and Hearing Sciences and my mentor, who has always supported me in every academic mission.

Again, many thanks to you all!

Jayanti Ray

Contents

The Building Blocks of Our Nervous System

OUTLINE

Neuron

Neuronal Functions

Supporting Cells

Clinical Notes

Review Questions
  Multiple Choice
  Fill in the Blanks

NEURON

The basic unit of life is the cell. The tissues that compose the nervous system are enormously complex. They are built of specialized cells called neurons that serve as structural and functional units in the nervous system. Neurons conduct nerve messages, process sensory information, compute appropriate behavioral responses, and signal what the body is to do. Through various modes of nerve conductions, nerve cells serve all sensorimotor activities as well as higher level functions such as speech, language, and cognition.

Each neuron has a cell body, dendrites, and an axon. The dendrites are thread-like processes that arise from the cell body. Dendrites receive impulses from other cells and carry them toward the cell body or axon. Axons are highly specialized long processes that extend from the cell body and conduct nerve impulses away from the cell body. Axons are covered with myelin sheaths, and bundles of myelin-coated axons comprise nerve fibers. The thicker the axon's myelin sheaths are, the faster is the propagation of the nerve impulse. Gaps between continuous myelin sheaths are called nodes of Ranvier. Any site of contact between an axon and a muscle fiber is called a neuromuscular junction.

Each axon divides into branches called telodendria. Within these telodendria is a swelling called the synaptic knob. The synaptic knob contains many tiny, smooth, hollow spheres and membranes called synaptic vesicles. Axonal synaptic vesicles contain chemical substances called neurotransmitters that help generate the action potential. Neurotransmitters may be either excitatory or inhibitory. If they are excitatory, activity is produced; if they are inhibitory, inactivity results.

The synapse is a point of connection between neurons, where the axon of one neuron contacts the dendrites of another. The synapse is composed of the synaptic knob and the plasma membrane of the adjacent neuron. Various portions of a cell can be involved in a synapse. Connections can be termed axodendritic, axosomatic, axoaxonic, or axosynaptic, depending on whether the synapse is with dendrites, the cell body, axons, or synapses of other cells. The gap between the synaptic knob and the postsynaptic membrane is called the synaptic cleft (Figures 1-1 to 1-3; Table 1-1).

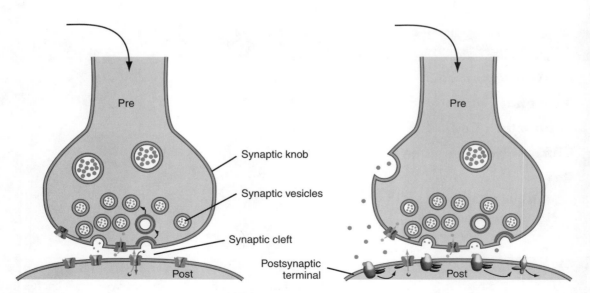

Figure 1-1   Structures at the synaptic level. (From Nolte J: *The human brain: an introduction to its functional anatomy,* ed 5, St Louis, 2002, Mosby.)

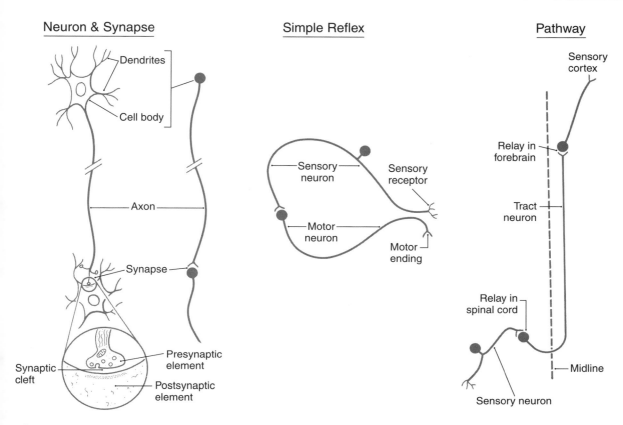

Figure 1-2   Types of synapses. (From Haines DE: *Fundamental neuroscience,* ed 2, Philadelphia, 2002, Churchill Livingstone.)

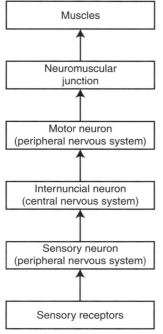

Figure 1-3   The sensorimotor pathway.

TABLE 1-1	Neuron Types, Locations, and Functions

Types of neurons	Location	Functions
Multipolar neurons have at least two processes: the axon and multiple dendrites	Central nervous system, e.g., spinal interneurons	Control motor, sensory, and integration of motor and sensory activities
Bipolar neurons have one dendrite and one axon	Special sensory receptors, e.g., retina of the eye, olfactory nerves, vestibulocochlear nerve	Carry sensory information
Unipolar neurons have a single process	Ganglia of the peripheral nervous system	Carry sensory information

NEURONAL FUNCTIONS

Neurons are classified according to function as sensory or motor. Sensory neurons (also called somatic afferent neurons) perceive sensations such as pain, temperature, and touch to the skin. General visceral afferent neurons receive sensory information from within the viscera (glands, organs, and membranes). General somatic efferent neurons innervate skeletal muscles, whereas general visceral efferent neurons provide motor innervation for smooth muscles, cardiac muscles, and glands. Special somatic afferent sensory neurons transmit the sensory messages linked to sight and hearing, while special visceral afferent sensory fibers transmit the sensory messages connected to smell and taste.

According to axonal length, neurons are classified as either Golgi I or Golgi II neurons. Golgi I cells have long axons and form various sensory and motor tracts. Golgi II cells, which have short axons, form interneurons, which conduct impulses from a sensory neuron to a motor neuron.

Adequate stimulation of the dendrites leads to the generation of an action potential at the axon hillock, the portion of the cell body from which the axon extends. The action potential results when there is adequate depolarization (increase of voltage when the inside of a neuron is positive) at the axon hillock. The wave propagated by the action potential is called a nerve impulse. The nerve impulse maintains the same action potential throughout the axon's length. When the action potential reaches the synaptic knob, synaptic vesicles are activated. These vesicles move to the plasma membrane of the synaptic knob where neurotransmitters are released into the synaptic cleft.

SUPPORTING CELLS

The glial cells in the nervous system function like glue and provide structural support for neurons. They also help provide nutrition, support, and insulation to the neurons. Glial cells are of three types:

1. Astrocytes
2. Microglia
3. Oligodendrocytes

Astrocytes are star-shaped cells that support neurons. Found in both gray and white matter, they help in neuronal and carbohydrate metabolism and aid in repairing the blood-brain barrier. Microglial cells are responsible for immune reactions in the nervous system. They help form scar tissues and thus protect cells from damage. They are also called the scavengers of the central nervous system (CNS). In the CNS, oligodendrocytes wrap around axons, producing myelin sheaths similar to the way Schwann cells function in the peripheral nervous system.

Ependymal cells are also considered a type of supporting cell in the CNS. They provide a lining for the ventricular cavities, which contain cerebrospinal fluid.

During cerebrovascular accidents, astrocytes and microglial cells proliferate and migrate to the site of the lesion. Microglial cells act as phagocytes and engulf the cellular debris. Astrocytes isolate the site of the damage from areas where there are healthy cells. In addition, they form glial scars to fill the site of lesion.

CLINICAL NOTES

- The process of myelin formation has a significant impact on the development of sensorimotor activities and cognition. If myelin maturation is delayed, various developmental disorders may result.
- Wallerian degeneration refers to the disintegration of the axon at the distal end, which occurs when the axon is injured. Axons degenerate before their myelin sheaths, and eventually the myelin sheaths start showing disintegration.
- If the nervous system is injured, glial cells increase in size and multiply in numbers.
- In multiple sclerosis, CNS myelin breaks.

Review Questions

I. Multiple Choice

1. The parts of the neuron that release neurotransmitters into the synaptic cleft is called the

   _____ .
   a. postsynaptic terminal
   b. presynaptic terminal
   c. axon hillock

2. Gaps in the myelin sheath are called _____ .
   a. synaptic gaps
   b. nodes of Ranvier
   c. axonic gaps

3. Fatty materials surrounding the axons are called _____ .
   a. myelin sheaths
   b. astrocyte sheaths
   c. microglial membranes

4. Myelin sheaths that cover the axons of neurons are designed for _____ .
   a. faster transport of neural impulses
   b. slower transport of neural impulses
   c. maintaining resting potential

5. The greater the diameter of the nerve fiber, the _____ is the conduction of the nerve impulse.
   a. slower
   b. faster

6. The _____ takes information away from the cell body.
   a. dendrite
   b. axon
   c. axon sheath

7. The _____ takes information to the cell body.
   a. dendrite
   b. axon
   c. axon sheath

8. The neural impulse travels in the following manner: _____ .
   a. motor neuron; sensory neuron; interneuron
   b. sensory neuron; interneuron; motor neuron
   c. interneuron; sensory neuron; motor neuron

9. Neurotransmitters that are released through the _____ neurons enter into the synaptic cleft to reach the receptor sites in the dendrites of _____ neurons.
   a. postsynaptic; presynaptic
   b. presynaptic; postsynaptic
   c. neither of the above

10. A neural impulse that carries information along neurons is called a/an _____ _____ .
    a. resting potential
    b. action potential
    c. membrane potential

11. The two types of cells in the nervous system are _____ and _____ _____ .
    a. white cells and gray cells
    b. glial cells and gray cells
    c. neurons and glial cells

12. _____ are specialized for nerve impulse conduction and are therefore responsible for most of the functional characteristics of nervous tissue.
    a. Neurons
    b. Glial cells
    c. Ependymal cells

13. _____ are typically short branching processes that form a major part of the cell's receptive area.
    a. Axons
    b. Dendrites
    c. Cell bodies

14. The central nervous system consists of gray and white matter. _____ form the gray matter and _____ form the white matter.
    a. Cell bodies; axons
    b. Axons; cell bodies
    c. Synapses; axons

15. Two neurons are separated by a narrow gap called a _____ .
    a. perikaryon
    b. neuropil
    c. synaptic cleft

16. The arrival of an impulse at an excitatory synapse causes _____ of the postsynaptic membrane, whereas the arrival of an impulse at an inhibitory synapse causes _____ .
    a. hyperpolarization; depolarization
    b. depolarization; hyperpolarization
    c. neither of the above

17. Axons terminate by branching into smaller sections, _____ , which include synaptic knobs at their ends.
    a. boutons
    b. telodendria
    c. synapses

18. _____ provide skeletal support to the brain cells and their processes. They protect the brain cells by contributing to the blood-brain barrier, which restricts the movement of certain substances in the blood to the brain.
    a. Microglial cells
    b. Ependymal cells
    c. Astrocytes

19. A neuron with no dendrites and a single axon is called a _____ neuron.
    a. unipolar
    b. bipolar
    c. multipolar

20. A bipolar neuron is _____ in nature.
    a. sensory
    b. motor
    c. sensorimotor

21. A _____ results from a change in electrochemical difference between the outside and inside of the cell membrane.
    a. process of repolarization
    b. nerve impulse
    c. resting potential

22. When the nerve impulse travels from one neuron to the other, the process is called _____ .
    a. temporal summation
    b. repolarization
    c. synaptic transmission

23. Endings of the axon have filament-like extensions called telodendria that end in a small round enlargement called a _____ .
    a. mitochondria
    b. vesicle
    c. synaptic knob

24. _____ contain neurochemical substances called neurotransmitters.
    a. Synaptic vesicles
    b. Presynaptic membranes
    c. Postsynaptic membranes

25. _____ produces depolarization of the postsynaptic membrane.
    a. GABA
    b. Acetylcholine
    c. Dopamine

26. Depolarization of the postsynaptic membrane is known as _____ postsynaptic potential, whereas hyperpolarization of the postsynaptic membrane is called _____ postsynaptic potential.
    a. inhibitory; excitatory
    b. excitatory; inhibitory
    c. neither of the above

27. _____ is the additive effect of impulses over time from the postsynaptic neuron to the other neurons.
    a. Spatial summation
    b. Temporal summation
    c. Excitatory summation

28. When a larger area of the axon acts on a cell body to continue the flow of impulse to succeeding neurons, it is called _____ .
    a. spatial summation
    b. temporal summation
    c. excitatory summation

29. _____ and _____ regulate basal ganglia motor functions.
    a. Peptides; norepinephrine
    b. Norepinephrine; serotonin
    c. Acetylcholine; dopamine

30. Antibodies interfere with the action of acetylcholine on muscle cells at the myoneural junction in a condition called _____ .
    a. multiple sclerosis
    b. myasthenia gravis
    c. cerebellar degeneration

31. Deficient cholinergic projections in the hippocampus and frontal cortex are found in a degenerative condition called _____ .
    a. Wilson's disease
    b. Alzheimer's disease
    c. multiple sclerosis

32. Reduced production and transmission of dopamine, associated with the degeneration of substantia nigra, are found in a condition called _____ .
    a. myasthenia gravis
    b. Parkinson's disease
    c. Alzheimer's disease

33. When there is a loss of GABA-producing neurons in the basal ganglia, a condition called

_____ results.
   a. Parkinson's disease
   b. Huntington's disease
   c. multiple sclerosis

II. Fill in the Blanks

Provide one-line definitions for each of the following terms.

1. Resting potential _____

2. Depolarization _____

3. Hyperpolarization _____

4. Neurotransmitters _____

5. Glial cells _____

6. Nodes of Ranvier _____

7. Myelination _____

8. Synapse _____

9. Wallerian degeneration _____

10. Axon _____

Answers to Review Questions

I Multiple Choice

1. b	6. b	10. b	14. a	18. c	22. c	26. b	30. b
2. b	7. a	11. c	15. c	19. a	23. c	27. b	31. b
3. a	8. b	12. a	16. b	20. a	24. a	28. a	32. b
4. a	9. b	13. b	17. b	21. b	25. b	29. c	33. b
5. b							

II. Fill in the Blanks

1. Resting potential: During this stage the neuron does not generate any action potential.

2. Depolarization: During this stage, intracellular potentials change to more positive values, indicating the onset of an action potential.

3. Hyperpolarization: During this stage, intracellular potentials change to a more negative value, indicating the end of an action potential.

4. Neurotransmitters: Excitatory or inhibitory neurochemical substances released at the synapses to alter the states of action potentials.

5. Glial cells: Supporting cells of the nervous system that have many functions, such as phagocytosis, nutrition, and myelin formation.

6. Nodes of Ranvier: Places along the axon where there is no myelin.

7. Myelination: Process of covering axons of neurons with fatty substances (myelin).

8. Synapse: Site of contact between one neuron and another neuron or the cells of a muscle or gland.

9. Wallerian degeneration: Fatty degenerative process that occurs at the distal end of the axon fragments when an axon is disconnected from the cell body of a neuron, the distal end of the axon fragments demonstrates a process called Wallerian degeneration.

10. Axon: Unbranched process of the nerve cell that helps in conducting an action potential.

2

Overview of the Nervous System

OBJECTIVES

After completing this chapter, the learner will:

- **Have a basic understanding of the complex architecture of the human nervous system.**
- **Know that the human nervous system is the most complex and highly organized system in the body.**
- **Understand various neurological disorders by knowing the nervous system's normal functions.**

DIVISIONS OF THE NERVOUS SYSTEM

Anatomically, the human nervous system is divided into the central and peripheral nervous systems (Figure 2-1). The central nervous system (CNS) consists of the brain and spinal cord, whereas the peripheral nervous system (PNS) is formed by 12 pairs of cranial and 31 pairs of spinal nerves. The human brain and cranial nerves are discussed in other chapters. The spinal cord is a long segment extending from the brain that includes paired spinal nerves. Each nerve has a dorsal sensory root and a ventral motor root (Figure 2-2).

Functionally, the nervous system has two divisions: the somatic and autonomic nervous systems. The somatic nervous system innervates muscles, skin, and mucous membranes, whereas the autonomic nervous system controls the activities of the smooth muscles, visceral glands, and blood vessels.

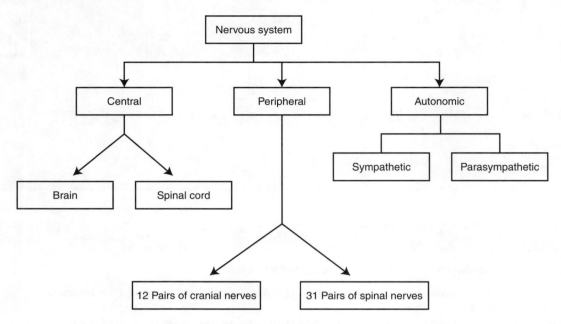

Figure 2-1   Divisions of the nervous system.

AUTONOMIC NERVOUS SYSTEM

The autonomic nervous system is also called the visceral system because it exerts control over the viscera of the body, including the cardiac muscles and various glands. The functions that are governed are purely motor. As the motor or efferent projections of the autonomic nervous system do not directly innervate the visceral organs, the outflow of autonomic nervous system is based on a two-neuron motor pathway. The first neuron is called preganglionic neuron whose axon is myelinated. The second neuron is called postganglionic neuron whose axon is partially myelinated. The cell body of the first neuron is located in the CNS (brain or spinal cord), whereas the cell body of the second neuron is located in one of the autonomic ganglia, all of which lie outside the CNS. The fibers of the second neuron or the postganglionic neuron actually terminate on specific visceral organs.

The autonomic nervous system is divided into two parts: the sympathetic and parasympathetic nervous systems. The sympathetic nervous system helps a person cope with stressful situations. It automatically sets the body for "fight" or "flight" by constricting the blood vessels, dilating the pupils, increasing the heart rate, elevating the body temperature, etc. The parasympathetic nervous system, on the other hand, prepares the body for relaxation by slowing down the heart rate, constricting the pupils, reducing the respiratory rate, etc. Both sympathetic and parasympathetic nervous systems are based on a two-neuron motor pathway. These systems innervate many organs of the body where their antagonistic actions serve to balance function and maintain homeostasis.

CLINICAL NOTES (FOCUSED ON THE PERIPHERAL NERVOUS SYSTEM)

- Spinal cord disorders include degenerative disorders of the spine (e.g., changes in the intervertebral disc and cervical spondylosis), thoracic disc disease, spinal stenosis, rheumatoid arthritis of the spine, spinal epidural abscess, spinal tumors, spinal cysts, and spinal arachnoiditis.

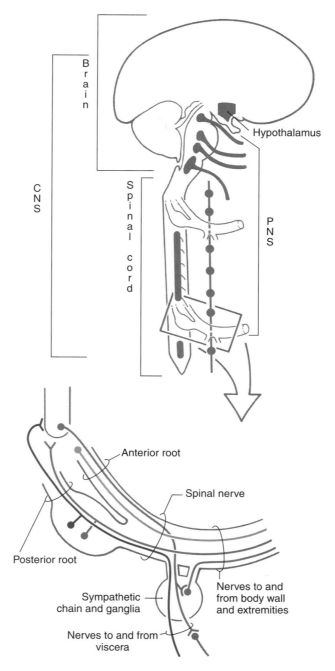

Figure 2-2   Peripheral nervous system consisting of the spinal cord and nerves. (From Haines DE: *Fundamental neuroscience,* ed 2, Philadelphia, 2002, Churchill Livingstone.)

- Myelitis is a disease caused by intrinsic demyelination and/or inflammation of the spinal cord. It can cause limb weakness of varying severity. This disease also produces a patch of numbness or tingling on a limb.
- Shy-Drager syndrome is a progressive disorder of the CNS and autonomic nervous system. Characteristics include postural hypotension, bradykinesia, tremors, balance problems, generalized weakness, double vision, speech impairments, and problems involving respirations, swallowing, and cardiac function.
- Guillain-Barre syndrome is a neurological disorder, evidencing damage to the peripheral nervous system. Varying degrees of weakness, abnormal sensations in the upper body, and cardiac problems are typically seen.
- Pain in the spine and nerve root pain may indicate the presence of malignant disease in the spine. Segmental neurological signs include lower motor neuron weakness, loss of deep tendon reflex, and abnormalities of dermatome sensory abilities.
- Myasthenia gravis is an autoimmune disease of the neuromuscular junction characterized by abnormal functioning of the acetylcholine receptors at the postsynaptic muscle membrane. Clinical signs and symptoms include fatigue, diplopia, ptosis, dysphagia, dysarthria, and facial weakness.
- Causalgia is damage to a peripheral nerve by a penetrating wound, which may result in an incapacitating disorder. There is severe pain in the affected limb along with skin changes.
- In peripheral neuropathy the pathological processes diffusely involve the peripheral nerves. The motor, sensory, and autonomic fibers can be affected uniformly or in isolation. Symptoms include symmetrical, distal motor, and sensory deficits.

Review Questions

I. Multiple Choice

1. The human nervous system is grossly divided into the central nervous system and the
   _____ nervous system.
   a. sympathetic
   b. autonomous
   c. peripheral

2. The central nervous system consists of _____ and _____ .
   a. cortex; subcortex
   b. cranial nerves; spinal cord
   c. parasympathetic ganglion; cerebrum
   d. brain; spinal cord

3. The functions of the cerebrum include all of the following except _____ .
   a. perception of sensory stimuli
   b. regulation of behaviors
   c. regulation of cognition and language
   d. regulation of vital function in the body, e.g., respiration
   e. mediation of reflexes

4. The _____ encloses and protects the brain.
   a. vertebrae
   b. cranium
   c. spinal column

5. The _____ provide(s) the bony structure of the spinal column.
   a. spinal nerves
   b. cranium
   c. vertebrae

6. The space inside the skull is called the _____ , which accommodates the
   soft tissues of the brain.
   a. vertebral column
   b. cranial vault
   c. foramen magnum

7. The brain is subdivided into cerebrum, brainstem, cerebellum, and _____ .
   a. ventricles
   b. spinal cord
   c. basal ganglia
   d. none of the above

8. The brainstem consists of midbrain, _____ , and _____ .
   a. basal ganglia; cerebellum
   b. thalamus; hypothalamus
   c. pons; medulla oblongata

9. Gray matter forms the _____ , whereas white matter forms the subcortex.
   a. motor nerve tracts
   b. sensory nerve tracts
   c. cerebral cortex

10. The white matter of the spinal cord consists of _____ .
    a. medial, superior, and inferior columns
    b. dorsal, lateral, and ventral columns
    c. superior, inferior, and rostral columns

11. The connections, or pathways, between groups of neurons in the central nervous system
    form bundles of nerve fibers or tracts and are called _____ .
    a. decussations
    b. fasciculi
    c. funiculi

12. Nerve fiber tracts present in the spinal cord are referred to as _____ .
    a. commissures
    b. fasciculi
    c. funiculi

13. The nervous system is constructed with _____ , meaning the right and
    left cerebral hemispheres are structurally symmetrical.
    a. unilateral organization
    b. bilateral symmetry
    c. principles of decussation
    d. none of the above

14. The right cerebral hemisphere receives information about the left side of the body and
    vice-versa. This is called _____ in our nervous system.
    a. crossed representation
    b. asymmetry
    c. uncrossed representation
    d. none of the above

15. The peripheral nervous system consists of the following:
    a. sensory receptors and motor endings
    b. sensory receptors, motor endings, and ganglia
    c. sensory receptors, motor endings, ganglia, and spinal nerves

16. The _____ are swellings on the dorsal roots of spinal nerves situated in the intervertebral formina, just proximal to the union of the dorsal and ventral roots that forms the spinal nerves.
    a. autonomic endings
    b. spinal ganglia
    c. autonomic ganglia

17. _____ include those of the sympathetic trunks along the sides of the vertebral bodies.
    a. Autonomic endings
    b. Autonomic ganglia
    c. Neither of the above

18. Peripheral nerves are arranged in bundles or _____ .
    a. fasciculi
    b. fibers
    c. tracts

19. The peripheral and cranial nerves contain nerve fibers that conduct information to the

    _____ .
    a. central nervous system
    b. spinal cord only
    c. neither of the above

20. There are _____ pairs of spinal or peripheral nerves.
    a. 12
    b. 31
    c. 15

21. Each segment of the spinal cord consists of two roots on each side: one dorsal and one

    _____ .
    a. medial
    b. ventral
    c. lateral

22. A dorsal root is _____ in nature, whereas a ventral root is

    _____ in nature.
    a. motor; sensory
    b. sensory; motor
    c. neither of the above

23. The _____ roots constitute motor outflow tracts from the spinal cord.
    a. dorsal
    b. ventral
    c. dorsal and ventral

24. The _____ roots, which are sensory in nature, contain afferent fibers from the nerve cell in the ganglion.
    a. ventral
    b. dorsal
    c. dorsal and ventral

25. The sensory component of each spinal nerve is distributed to a _____ .
    a. visceral afferent area
    b. dermatome
    c. myotome
    d. none of the above

26. _____ refers to the skeletal musculature innervated by motor axons in a given spinal root.
    a. Myotome
    b. Dermatome
    c. Visceral efferent area

27. A common peripheral neuromuscular disorder is _____ .
    a. peripheral neuropathy
    b. motor neuron disease
    c. myasthenia gravis
    d. muscle disease
    e. all of the above

28. Motor neuron disease is characterized by all of the following except _____
    _____ .
    a. generalized weakness of muscles
    b. involvement of bulbar muscle
    c. upper motor neuron signs and symptoms
    d. sensory symptoms

29. Peripheral neuropathy is characterized by all of the following except _____
    _____ .
    a. distal wasting and weakness of the muscles
    b. distal sensory signs and symptoms
    c. bulbar involvement
    d. none of the above

30. Muscle disease is characterized by all of the following except _____ .
    a. muscle weakness
    b. involvement of distal muscles
    c. muscle wasting

31. When the sympathetic nervous system acts, the following reactions take place:
    a. faster heart beat
    b. rapid, deep breathing
    c. cold skin
    d. dilated pupils
    e. all of the above

32. When the parasympathetic nervous system acts, the following reactions take place:
    a. low blood pressure
    b. low heart rate
    c. low respiratory rate
    d. constricted pupils
    e. all of the above

II. Fill in the Blanks

Explain the following terms pertaining to various nervous systems.

1. Peripheral nerves: _____

2. Sensory receptors: _____

3. Ganglia: _____

4. Motor endings: _____

5. Cranial nerves: _____

6. Preganglionic neuron: _____

7. Postganglionic neuron: _____

8. Sympathetic trunk: _____

9. Brain: _____

10. Thoracolumbar flow: _____

11. Spinal cord: _____

Answers to Review Questions

I. Multiple Choice

1. c	5. c	9. c	13. b	17. a	21. b	25. b	29. c
2. d	6. b	10. b	14. a	18. a	22. b	26. a	30. b
3. e	7. c	11. b	15. c	19. a	23. b	27. e	31. e
4. b	8. c	12. c	16. c	20. b	24. b	28. d	32. e

II. Fill in the Blanks

1. Peripheral nerves: Also called spinal nerves; denotes nerves that belong to the peripheral nervous system.

2. Sensory receptors: Specialized nerve endings that respond to sensory stimuli (touch, temperature, pain, pressure, etc.) in the environment.

3. Ganglia: An aggregation of nerve cell bodies located in the peripheral nervous system.

4. Motor endings: Ends of motor neurons that branch off of the axon to make synapses with muscles.

5. Cranial nerves: Nerves that emerge from, or enter the cranium, and form a part of the peripheral nervous system. There are 12 pairs of cranial nerves that mediate various motor, sensory, and visceral functions.

6. Preganglionic neuron: Myelinated neuron situated proximal to an autonomic ganglion; refers to motor neurons in the autonomic nervous system that have a cell body in the brainstem and spinal cord.

7. Postganglionic neuron: Unmyelinated neuron originating from cells in an autonomic ganglion; both preganglionic and postganglionic neurons form a two-neuron pathway in the autonomic nervous system.

8. Sympathetic trunk: Division of the autonomic nervous system that prepares the body for fight or flight during a stressful situation.

9. Brain: Mass consisting of gray and white matter; a division of the central nervous system, which helps in sensorimotor innervation of the body.

10. Thoracolumbar flow: Outflow of the sympathetic nervous system that is located in the lateral gray horn of the spinal cord between the thoracic and lumbar segments; also called sympathetic chain.

11. Spinal cord: A cylindrical structure, which is a part of the central nervous system. It is a caudal continuation of the medulla oblongata surrounded by meninges. It helps integrate sensorimotor information.

3

A Tour of the Human Brain: Part I

OBJECTIVES

After completing this chapter, the learner will:

- **Know the major divisions of the brain and lobes of the cerebral cortex.**
- **Understand how the brain functions as part of the central nervous system.**

OUTLINE

Major Divisions of the Brain

Cerebral Hemispheres
Basal Ganglia, Thalamus, and Hypothalamus
Brainstem
Cerebellum

Lobes of the Brain

Clinical Notes

Review Questions

Multiple Choice
Fill in the Blanks: Brain
Fill in the Blanks: Cerebellar lesions
Fill in the Blanks: Lesions in basal ganglia
Matching

MAJOR DIVISIONS OF THE BRAIN (FIGURE 3-1)

As outlined in Chapter 2, the human nervous system is broadly divided into central and peripheral nervous systems, with the central nervous system (CNS) consisting of the brain and the spinal cord and the peripheral nervous system (PNS) consisting of the peripheral nerves (cranial

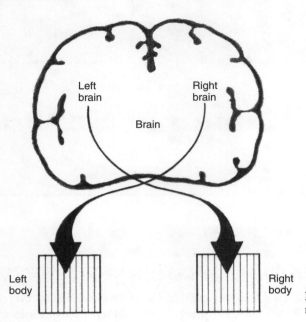

Figure 3-1   Contralateral innervation of motor control by the cortex.

nerves and spinal nerves), sensory receptors, and motor endings. The human brain has four main divisions, as follows:

1. Cerebral hemispheres
2. Basal ganglia, thalamus, and hypothalamus
3. Brainstem
4. Cerebellum

Cerebral Hemispheres

The cerebral hemispheres are two large structures separated from each other by the median longitudinal fissure. The outer surface of the cerebral hemispheres, the cortex, is composed of gray matter. The cortex has convolutions called gyri. Gyri are separated by shallow grooves called sulci and deeper grooves called fissures. Each hemisphere is divided into four major lobes (frontal, parietal, temporal, and occipital) (Figure 3-2), and they are bounded by lateral and central fissures.

The right and left cerebral hemispheres are separated by the corpus callosum (Figure 3-3), which works like a bridge, allowing information to pass from one side of the brain to the other (Figures 3-4 and 3-5). The cerebrum is interconnected by fibers that are generally of three types: (1) association fibers connect various areas within the cerebral hemispheres; (2) commissural fibers (e.g., corpus callosum) connect the two hemispheres; and (3) projection fibers connect the cerebrum to lower centers of the CNS. They are either afferent or efferent.

Basal Ganglia, Thalamus, and Hypothalamus (Figure 3-6)

The basal ganglia consist of masses of gray matter deep within the cerebral hemispheres. These structures have control over movements and posture. The basal ganglia function to adjust the body to perform desirable movements and help inhibit unwanted movements. Damage to the basal ganglia leads to movement disorders. The motor cortex and thalamus form the main loop that helps the basal ganglia work. Information is sent from the motor cortex to the basal ganglia and is relayed back via the thalamus.

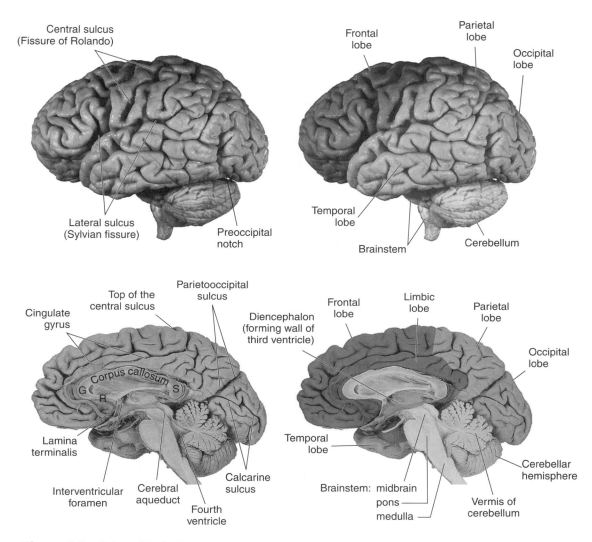

Figure 3-2 Lobes of the brain. (From Nolte J: *The human brain: an introduction to its functional anatomy,* ed 5, St Louis, 2002, Mosby.)

The three major parts of the basal ganglia are as follows:
1. Caudate nucleus
2. Putamen
3. Globus pallidus

Together the putamen and the globus pallidus are called the lentiform nucleus (Figure 3-7). The putamen is the lateral portion of the lentiform nucleus, and the globus pallidus is the medial region. The lentiform nucleus and the caudate nucleus are together called the corpus striatum. The corpus striatum is a large mass of gray matter with motor functions situated near the base of each hemisphere. The basal ganglia are a part of the extrapyramidal system, and they interact with the cerebral cortex via various loops in all motor activities.

The thalamus is a large rounded structure consisting of gray matter. It looks like two egg-shaped masses lying on either side of the third ventricle. The thalamus is a relay center for sensory stimuli and consists of several regions of cell bodies (gray matter). The thalamus receives sensory input from the body and conveys the same to sensory areas of the cerebral cortex. The

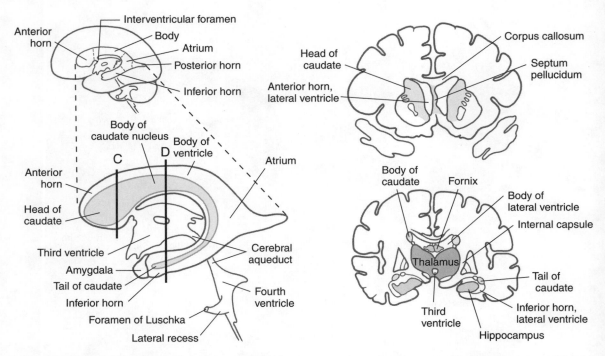

Figure 3-3   Corpus callosum. (From Haines DE: *Fundamental neuroscience,* ed 2, Philadelphia, 2002, Churchill Livingstone.)

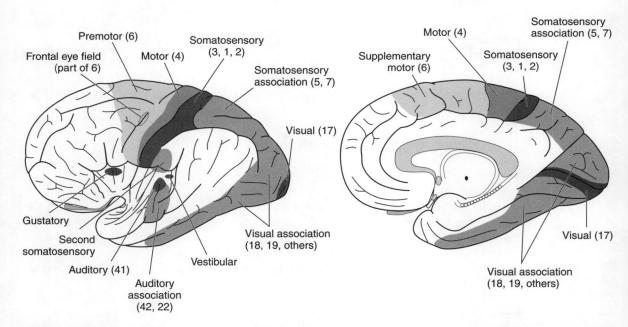

Figure 3-4   Sensory and motor areas of the brain. (Modified from von Economo C: *The cytoarchitectonics of the human cerebral cortex,* Oxford, 1929, Oxford University Press.)

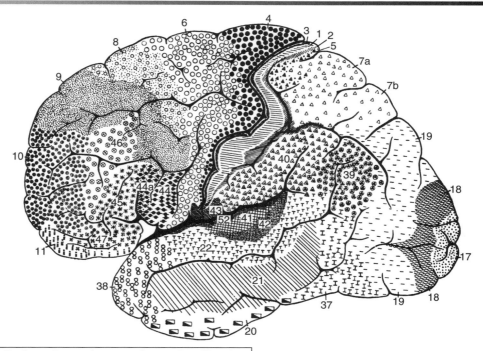

Brodmann's areas important for speech and hearing

3, 1, 2: Primary sensory areas or postcentral gyrus

5, 7, 39, 40: Secondary sensory areas

39: Angular gyrus

40: Supramarginal gyrus

44: Broca's area

41, 42: Primary auditory areas or Heschl's gyrus

22: Secondary auditory area or Wernicke's area

4: Primary motor area or precentral gyrus

6: Premotor area

8: Prefrontal area

17: Primary visual area

18, 19: Secondary visual areas

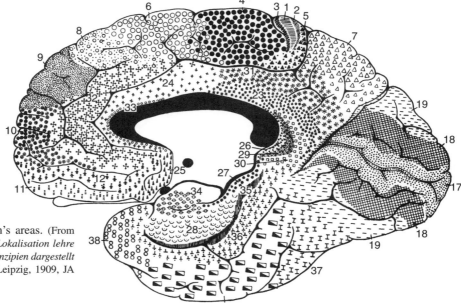

Figure 3-5 Brodmann's areas. (From Brodmann K: *Vergleichende Lokalisation lehre der Grosshirnrinde in ihren Prinzipien dargestellt auf Grund des Zellenbaues,* Leipzig, 1909, JA Barth.)

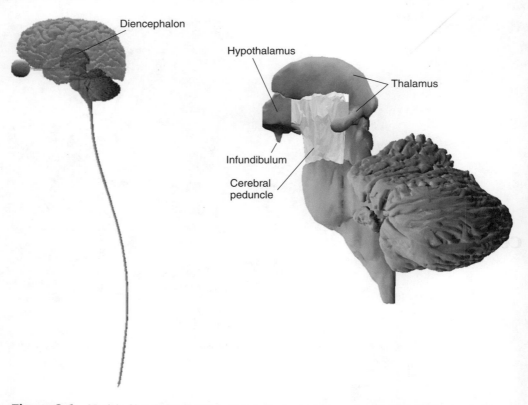

Figure 3-6   Nuclei of basal ganglia. (From Nolte J: *The human brain: an introduction to its functional anatomy,* ed 5, St Louis, 2002, Mosby.)

epithalamus includes small tracts and nuclei, together with the pineal body, an endocrine organ. The hypothalamus is the principal autonomic center of the brain, which controls parasympathetic and sympathetic nervous systems. The subthalamus includes sensory tracts that proceed to the thalamus; nerve fibers originating in the cerebellum and corpus striatum; and the subthalamic nucleus, a motor nucleus. The thalamus distributes sensory and motor information to the cortex and receives control information from the cortex. It also receives information from all of the senses except taste and smell, then organizes and routes the information to the appropriate cortical areas.

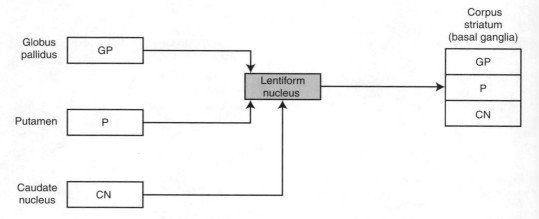

Figure 3-7   Thalamus and hypothalamus.

Brainstem

The brainstem, also called the bulb, is divided into the midbrain, pons, and medulla oblongata (Figure 3-8). The brainstem contains various cranial nerve nuclei, so that damage to certain areas of the brainstem produces cranial nerve disorders. Many ascending and descending tracts pass through various levels of the brainstem.

   The inferior and superior colliculi of the midbrain help mediate auditory and visual reflexes, respectively. The tectum of the midbrain helps in detecting reflexes. The medulla controls vital functions such as breathing, heart rate, and respiration. The reticular system is a group of neurons occupying most brainstem areas. This system functions in sleep, alertness, and consciousness. The reticular formation also helps in basic arousal and vital survival reflexes. Any damage to this system results in stupor and coma. Overall, damage to the brainstem leads to unconsciousness, coma, and possibly death.

Cerebellum

The cerebellum consists of the cerebellar cortex, two hemispheres, internal white matter, four pairs of nuclei, and three cerebellar peduncles. Each cerebellar hemisphere is divided into three lobes, the floccular, anterior, and posterior. Four nuclei (dentate, emboliform, globose, and fastigial) are embedded in the internal white matter. The dentate nucleus participates in limb movements and communicates with the basal ganglia and motor cortex. Emboliform and globose nuclei help regulate movements, and the fastigial nucleus is responsible for body

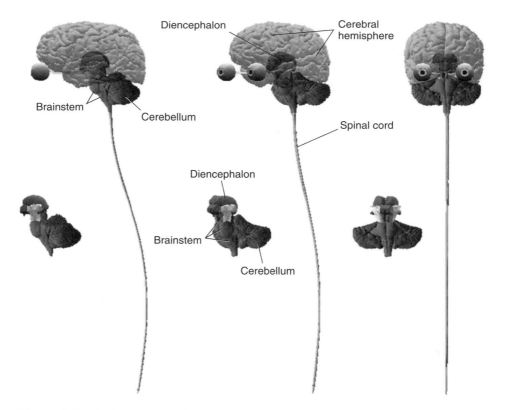

Figure 3-8   Brainstem, cerebellum, and cerebrum. (From Nolte J: *The human brain: an introduction to its functional anatomy,* ed 5, St Louis, 2002, Mosby.)

posture and equilibrium. The cerebellar peduncles connect the cerebellum to the various parts of the brain. The cerebellum is responsible for synergistic and coordinated movements of voluntary muscles. It is also responsible for maintaining muscle tone and body equilibrium and contributes to muscle synergy (coordination and smoothness in time and space), movement range, and strength.

LOBES OF THE BRAIN

Besides the four main lobes (Table 3-1), there exists another lobe, called the limbic lobe. It consists of the parahippocampal gyrus, subcallosal gyrus, and cingulate gyrus. This lobe is associated with various behaviors, emotions, and memory. The functions regulated by the limbic system include energy and water balance, automatic functions, endocrine functions, and sexual and emotional behaviors.

On the medial surface of the temporal lobe are located the amygdala and hippocampus. The amygdala is related to the autonomic nervous system. It is also linked to the frontal cortex in that it is involved with conscious emotional response to an event. Damage in the amygdala results in the loss of recognition of emotional responses. The hypothalamus and the brainstem autonomic centers are the output centers for the amygdala. The hippocampal nuclei are responsible for forming short-term memory and then help in conversion to long-term memory.

CLINICAL NOTES

Focal syndromes pertaining to the four major lobes are discussed here. The rest of the clinical notes are embedded in the questions that follow.

Focal frontal lobe syndrome:
* Mood and behavior problems
* Disinhibition and lack of concern
* Inability to perform complex mental tasks
* Poor concentration
* Lack of abstract thinking
* Presence of grasp reflex, suckling reflex, etc.

Focal temporal lobe syndrome:
* Memory deficits
* Learning difficulties

Focal parietal lobe syndrome:
* Gerstmann's syndrome (right-left disorientation, dyscalculia, dysgraphia, and finger agnosia)
* Constructional apraxia
* Visual or sensory neglect

TABLE 3-1	Main Lobes of the Brain and Their Functions

Lobes of the Brain	Functions
Frontal lobe	Higher-order executive functions, personality
Temporal lobe	Auditory processing and interpretation
Parietal lobe	Somatosensory information
Occipital lobe	Vision

Focal occipital lobe syndrome:
- Visual hallucinations
- Prosopagnosia (difficulty recognizing familiar faces)
- Achromatopia (loss of color perception)
- Visual disorientation
- Cortical blindness
- Anton's syndrome (denial of visual disability and confabulations)

Review Questions

I. Multiple Choice

1. The cerebrum constitutes _____ % of the total brain weight.
   a. 60
   b. 48
   c. 78

2. An average human brain weighs about _____ pounds and is 78% water.
   a. 6
   b. 3
   c. 8

3. The surface of the brain is characterized by swellings called _____ and

   ditches called _____ .
   a. sulci; gyri
   b. gyri; sulci
   c. neither of the above

4. A shallower ditch is called a _____ and a deeper ditch is called a

   _____ .
   a. fissure; sulcus
   b. sulcus; fissure
   c. gyrus; sulcus
   d. none of the above

5. The central fissure is also called the fissure of _____ .
   a. Sylvius
   b. Rolando
   c. Reil

6. The lateral fissure is also called the fissure of _____ .
   a. Sylvius
   b. Rolando
   c. Reil

7. There are two main fissures (deep grooves) in the brain: _____ and
   transverse.
   a. central
   b. horizontal
   c. longitudinal

8. There are three different sulci (shallow grooves) in the brain: _____ ,
   parieto-occipital, and lateral.
   a. central
   b. temporal
   c. occipital

9. The lower boundary of the frontal lobe is the _____ fissure and the
   posterior boundary is the _____ fissure.
   a. central; lateral
   b. lateral; central
   c. central; longitudinal

10. The precentral gyrus (motor strip) lies _____ to the central sulcus.
    a. anterior
    b. posterior
    c. superior

11. The postcentral gyrus (sensory strip) lies _____ to the central sulcus.
    a. anterior
    b. posterior
    c. superior

12. The outer layer of the brain is made up of _____ matter and the inner
    layer of the brain is made up of _____ matter.
    a. white; gray
    b. gray; white
    c. gray; gray

13. Each cerebral hemisphere communicates with the _____ side of the
    body.
    a. contralateral
    b. ipsilateral
    c. neither of the above

14. Visual areas are located in the _____ lobe.
    a. temporal
    b. parietal
    c. occipital

15. Auditory areas are located in the _____ lobe.
    a. temporal
    b. parietal
    c. occipital

16. The frontal lobes account for about _____ of the surface area of the
    brain.
    a. two thirds
    b. one third
    c. one half

17. The _____ lobe makes up approximately the bottom third of each hemisphere.
   a. occipital
   b. temporal
   c. frontal

18. The _____ lobe is a patch of the cortex that is folded into the lateral fissure.
   a. insular
   b. occipital
   c. thalamic

19. The cerebrum is involved with all of the following except _____ .
   a. voluntary movements
   b. vision
   c. memory
   d. reflexes

20. The _____ connects two cerebral hemispheres.
   a. arcuate fasciculus
   b. corpus striatum
   c. corpus callosum

21. The hypothalamus is involved with which of the following functions?
   a. Regulation of body temperature
   b. Water balance
   c. Metabolism
   d. All of the above

22. The _____ is involved with the production of normal and smooth coordinated movements.
   a. medulla oblongata
   b. midbrain
   c. cerebellum

23. The spinal cord is involved with the _____ .
   a. ascending pathways
   b. descending pathways
   c. reflex mechanism
   d. all of the above

24. The cerebral hemispheres are separated by a deep fissure called the _____ _____ fissure.
   a. lateral
   b. longitudinal
   c. central

25. According to the _____ _____ theory, certain neural functions are controlled by one hemisphere of the brain.
    a. cerebral suppression
    b. cerebral dominance
    c. neither of the above

26. The _____ is the integrator of bodily control and the main coordinator of movements.
    a. cerebellum
    b. cerebrum
    c. brainstem

27. The _____ connects the two hemispheres.
    a. corpus striatum
    b. corpus callosum
    c. arcuate fasciculus

28. The corpus callosum belongs to the _____ group of fibers.
    a. projection
    b. associative
    c. commissural

29. Areas 39 and 40 are present in the _____ lobe.
    a. temporal
    b. frontal
    c. neither of the above

30. Area 22 is also called _____ .
    a. Heschl's gyrus
    b. Wernicke's area
    c. neither of the above

31. Areas 44 and 45 are called _____ .
    a. Broca's area
    b. supramarginal gyrus
    c. angular gyrus

32. Areas 4, 6, and 8 constitute the _____ area.
    a. sensory
    b. motor
    c. sensorimotor

33. Areas 5 and 7 are present in the _____ lobe.
    a. frontal
    b. parietal
    c. neither of the above

34. The portions of the inferior parietal lobule that surround upturned ends of the lateral sulcus and superior temporal sulcus are called the _____ and _____ _____ gyrus, respectively.
    a. angular; supramarginal
    b. supramarginal; angular
    c. supramarginal; central

35. The corpus callosum may be viewed if the brain section is _____ .
    a. sagittal
    b. lateral
    c. neither of the above

36. Inferior and superior colliculi are present in the _____ .
    a. pons
    b. midbrain
    c. medulla oblongata

37. The _____ of the midbrain helps in mediating visual reflexes and in detecting movements.
    a. tectum
    b. tegmentum
    c. cerebral peduncles
    d. none of the above

38. The insular lobe is also called the _____ .
    a. island of Reil
    b. island of Sylvius
    c. island of Rolando

39. _____ is a dominant hereditary disorder that causes progressive degeneration of the corpus striatum.
    a. Cerebral palsy
    b. Huntington's chorea
    c. Hemiballismus

40. _____ causes muscular rigidity, tremor, slow shuffling gait, and a general lack of movement.
    a. Parkinson's disease
    b. Pick's disease
    c. Huntington's chorea

II. Fill in the Blanks

1. The _____ is known as the main sensory relay center for the nervous system.

2. The _____ is located below the thalamus, which controls the autonomous nervous system. It is also concerned with temperature control, water balance, emotional states, and control over the autonomic nervous system.

3. The _____ body in the thalamus is concerned with hearing and _____ _____ body in the thalamus is concerned with vision.

4. The _____ , _____ , and _____ form the brainstem. The brainstem contains nuclei of various cranial nerves.

5. The _____ of the midbrain comprises various motor and sensory tracts.

6. The crus cerebri (a pair of huge fiber bundles) is located in the _____ .

7. The _____ is located between the tegmentum and crus cerebri.

8. The _____ , _____ , and _____ make up the cerebral peduncle.

9. Two midbrain structures, called the _____ and the _____ _____ , are involved in motor control and muscle tension.

10. The _____ is considered the seat for consciousness.

11. The _____ is located under the occipital lobe.

12. The pons is separated from the cerebellum by a cavity containing cerebrospinal fluid that is called the fourth _____ .

13. The respiratory and cardiac centers are located in the _____ .

14. The important landmarks in the brainstem are called _____ (swellings) and olives (oval elevations).

15. A dense band of motor and sensory nerve fibers called the _____ passes through the thalamus and basal ganglia.

16. _____ and sensory disruptions almost always follow damage in the internal capsule.

17. All spinicerebellar fibers enter the _____ on the same side on which they entered the spinal cord.

18. Ventral and dorsal spinocerebellar tracts supply _____ impulses to the cerebellum.

19. The _____ nucleus of the cerebellum is part of the feedback mechanism to the vestibular nuclei, which then discharge to the lower motor neuron via lateral and medial vestibulospinal tracts.

III. Fill in the Blanks

Diagnose the following cerebellar lesions.

1. Excess loudness and uneven stress patterns in speech: _____

2. Floppy and weak muscles: _____

3. Jerky motor acts secondary to loss of coordination: _____

4. Inability to judge the distance: _____

5. Abnormal eye movements: _____

6. Inability to perform rapidly alternating movements: _____

7. Tremors during movements: _____

8. Loss of proper coordination between muscles; abnormal gait: _____

IV. Fill in the Blanks

Diagnose the following lesions related to the basal ganglia.

1. Relatively rapid, jerky, irregular, and unpredictable involuntary movements caused by a lesion in the contralateral caudate nucleus and putamen: _____

2. Involuntary, irregular, slow, and writhing movements caused by a lesion in the putamen:

   _____

3. Violent, involuntary movements of proximal joints caused by a lesion in the contralateral subthalamic nucleus: _____

4. Rhythmic, regular, and oscillating involuntary movements caused by lesions in the substantia nigra, red nucleus, cerebellum, and connections: _____

V. Matching

Match the structures of the brain to their functions.

1. Fornix	a. Auditory processing
2. Pons	b. Respiration
3. Medulla	c. Executive functioning
4. Thalamus	d. Somatosensory information
5. Occipital lobe	e. Aggressive behavior
6. Parietal lobe	f. Sleep
7. Frontal lobe	g. Vision
8. Temporal lobe	h. Relay center for sensory information

Answers to Review Questions

I. Multiple Choice

1. c	6. a	11. b	16. b	21. d	26. a	31. a	36. b
2. b	7. c	12. b	17. b	22. c	27. b	32. b	37. a
3. b	8. a	13. a	18. a	23. d	28. c	33. b	38. a
4. b	9. b	14. c	19. d	24. b	29. c	34. b	39. b
5. b	10. a	15. a	20. c	25. b	30. b	35. b	40. a

II. Fill in the Blanks

1. thalamus

2. hypothalamus

3. MGB, LGB(Medial Geniculate Body, Lateral Geniculate Body)

4. midbrain, pons, and medulla oblongata

5. tegmentum

6. midbrain

7. substantia nigra

8. tegmentum, crus cerebri, substantia nigra

9. red nucleus, substantia nigra

10. reticular formation

11. cerebellum

12. ventricle

13. pons

14. pyramids

15. internal capsule

16. Motor

17. cerebellum

18. proprioceptive

19. fastigial

III. Fill in the Blanks

1. ataxia

2. hypotonia

3. asynergia

4. dysmetria

5. nystagmus

6. adiadochokinesia

7. intention tremors

8. ataxia

IV. Fill in the Blanks

1. Huntington's chorea

2. athetosis

3. hemiballismus

4. tremor

V. Matching

1. e   2. f   3. b   4. h   5. g   6. d   7. c   8. a

4

A Tour of the Human Brain: Part II

OBJECTIVES

After completing this chapter, the learner will:

- Understand about meninges, the coverings of the brain and spinal cord.
- Know that ventricles carry cerebrospinal fluid and supply blood to the brain.
- Determine how these structures are related to neuropathological conditions.

OUTLINE

Meninges

Clinical Notes

Ventricles and the Cerebrospinal Fluid

Clinical Notes

Blood Supply to the Brain

Clinical Notes

Review Questions

Meninges

   Fill in the Blanks
   Multiple Choice
   True or False

The Ventricles and the Cerebrospinal Fluid

   Fill in the Blanks
   Multiple Choice

Blood Supply to the Brain

   Fill in the Blanks
   Matching
   Multiple Choice

MENINGES

The brain has a soft consistency and for protection it is housed in the bony cranial vault. Further protection is offered by surrounding membranous layers that are called meninges (Figure 4-1). The outermost layer is called dura mater, which is thicker than the middle and inner layers. The middle layer is called the arachnoid membrane, and the innermost layer is the pia mater. The pia mater is very thin and has a dense mesh of capillaries. The space between the skull and the dura mater is called the epidural space. The space between the dura mater and the arachnoid membrane is called the subdural space. The space between the arachnoid membrane and the pia mater is the subarachnoid space, which is filled with cerebrospinal fluid.

CLINICAL NOTES

- Meningitis is an infection of the fluid found in the spinal cord and surrounding the brain. Usually either a virus or a bacterium causes the infection. Viral meningitis is generally less severe and resolves without specific treatment, while bacterial meningitis can be quite severe and may result in brain damage, hearing loss, or learning disability. High fever, headache, and stiff neck are common symptoms of meningitis in anyone over age 2 years. These symptoms can develop over several hours, or they may take 1 to 2 days. Other symptoms can include nausea, vomiting, discomfort looking into bright lights, confusion, and sleepiness. In newborns and small infants the classic symptoms of fever, headache, and neck stiffness may be absent or difficult to detect, and the infant may only appear slow or inactive or be irritable. The infant may vomit or feed poorly. As the disease progresses, patients of any age may have seizures.
- Subdural hematomas are common during the birthing process. When a subdural hematoma presses on the brain, it causes dizziness, headaches, apathy, falling, confusion, and drowsiness.

VENTRICLES AND THE CEREBROSPINAL FLUID

There are four ventricles (Figure 4-2). Lateral ventricles are found in each cerebral hemisphere. The third ventricle is in the thalamus, and the medulla, pons, and cerebellum form the boundaries of the fourth ventricle. The ventricles carry a clear fluid called cerebrospinal fluid (CSF). CSF fills the entire subarachnoid space, which acts as a protective cushion around the brain and spinal cord. In each ventricle a structure called the choroid plexus produces CSF. The CSF from the lateral ventricles flows out via the interventricular foramen of Monroe and into the third ventricle, which is situated below and medial to the lateral ventricles. The fluid then flows into the narrow aqueduct of Sylvius (cerebral aqueduct) located in the midbrain (Figure 4-3). Then the liquid drains into the fourth ventricle in the area of the pons and medulla. From there, the cerebrospinal fluid fills the subarachnoid space (Figure 4-4).

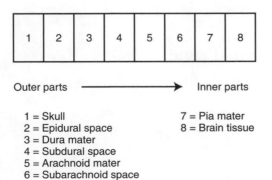

| 1 | 2 | 3 | 4 | 5 | 6 | 7 | 8 |

Outer parts ⟶ Inner parts

1 = Skull
2 = Epidural space
3 = Dura mater
4 = Subdural space
5 = Arachnoid mater
6 = Subarachnoid space

7 = Pia mater
8 = Brain tissue

Figure 4-1   The meninges.

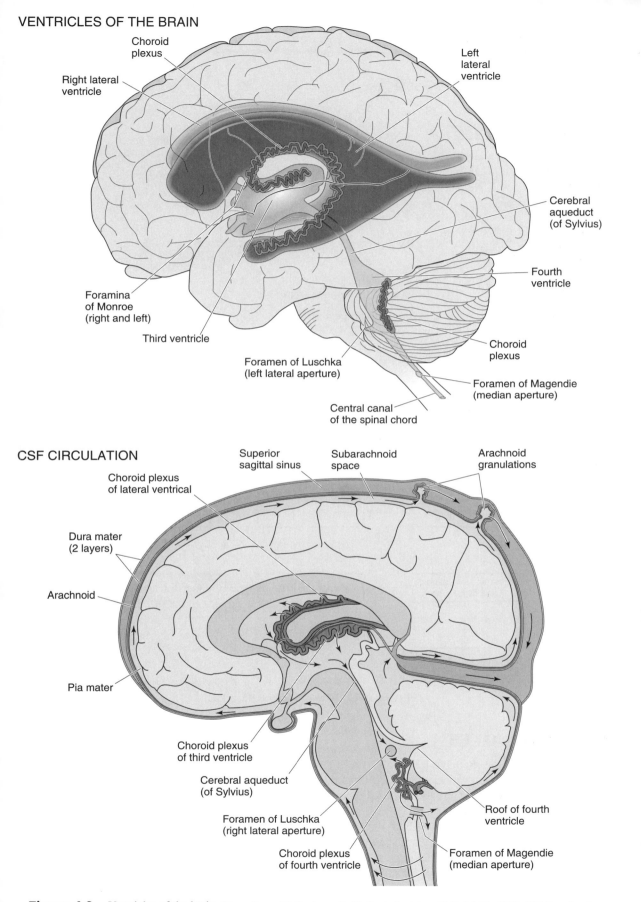

VENTRICLES OF THE BRAIN

Choroid plexus

Right lateral ventricle

Left lateral ventricle

Cerebral aqueduct (of Sylvius)

Foramina of Monroe (right and left)

Third ventricle

Foramen of Luschka (left lateral aperture)

Central canal of the spinal chord

Fourth ventricle

Choroid plexus

Foramen of Magendie (median aperture)

CSF CIRCULATION

Superior sagittal sinus

Subarachnoid space

Arachnoid granulations

Choroid plexus of lateral ventrical

Dura mater (2 layers)

Arachnoid

Pia mater

Choroid plexus of third ventricle

Cerebral aqueduct (of Sylvius)

Foramen of Luschka (right lateral aperture)

Choroid plexus of fourth ventricle

Roof of fourth ventricle

Foramen of Magendie (median aperture)

Figure 4-2   Ventricles of the brain. (From Boron W, Boulpaep E: *Medical physiology*, Philadelphia, 2003, WB Saunders.)

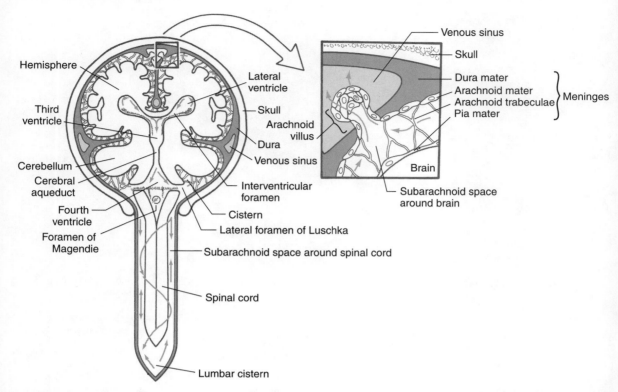

Figure 4-3   Ventricular system. (From Haines DE: *Fundamental neuroscience,* ed 2, Philadelphia, 2002, Churchill Livingstone.)

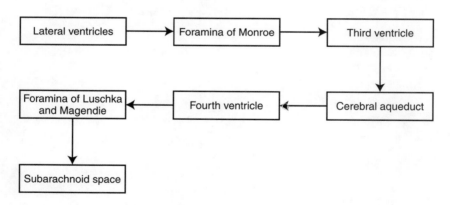

Figure 4-4   Flow of cerebrospinal fluid.

CLINICAL NOTES

- If the drainage pathways of CSF are obstructed at any point, the fluid accumulates in the ventricles inside the brain, causing them to swell and compress surrounding tissues. In newborns and infants, the head enlarges (hydrocephalus). In older children and adults the head size cannot increase because the bones that form the skull are completely joined together. The majority of infants born with spina bifida have hydrocephalus. In addition to the lesion in the spinal cord, there are abnormalities in the physical structure of certain parts of the brain that prevent proper drainage of CSF.

- Tumors, encephalitis, inadequate CSF resorption into the venous sinuses, and inadequacy of structures in the venous sinuses may cause increased intracranial pressure. Features of elevated intracranial pressure include a decrease in the level of consciousness, headache, vomiting, and papilledema.
- Encephalitis is a destructive inflammation of the brain substance that usually produces confusion, headaches, and seizures. Herpes simplex encephalitis is the commonest form of severe encephalitis.

BLOOD SUPPLY TO THE BRAIN

Two pairs of arteries, the vertebral arteries and the internal carotid arteries, supply blood to the brain. The vertebral arteries serve as the source for the anterior and posterior spinal arteries and the posterior inferior cerebellar artery. At the beginning of the pons, the basilar artery is formed by joining of two vertebral arteries (Figure 4-5, *A*). The posterior cerebral arteries arise from the basilar artery, which also gives rise to the anterior inferior cerebellar artery, pontine branches, labyrinthine arteries, and superior cerebellar arteries. The internal carotid artery enters the skull and feeds the anterior and middle cerebral arteries (Figure 4-5, *B*). From the middle cerebral artery the striate branch arises. Branches of the middle cerebral artery are found in the lateral fissure. The interhemispheric fissure contains branches of the anterior cerebral artery. The area of the brain where cerebral arteries overlap is called the watershed region. In an anastomotic ring known as the "circle of Willis" (Figures 4-6 and 4-7), the anterior cerebral arteries are connected via the anterior communicating arteries and the posterior communicating artery connects the middle cerebral artery with the posterior cerebral artery (Figure 4-8). If an artery is blocked, the blood supplies the designated area via detour pathways. This phenomenon is called collateral circulation.

CLINICAL NOTES

- The middle cerebral artery is the most direct and largest continuation of the internal carotid artery; therefore the incidence of emboli and metastases is higher in the territory of this vessel.
- Symptoms related to damage of the middle cerebral artery include dysphasia, dyslexia, dysgraphia, paralysis, and loss of sensation of the contralateral side of the face and upper limb.

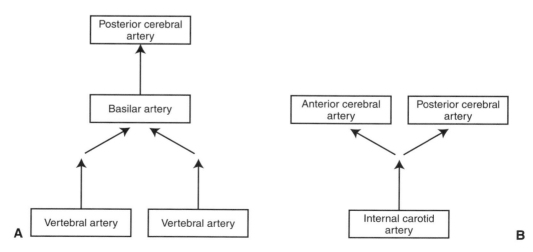

Figure 4-5 Branching of vertebral and internal carotid arteries.

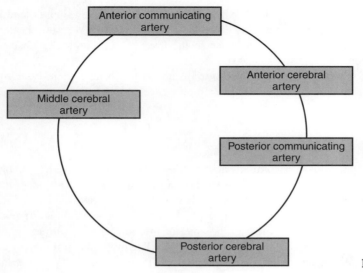

Figure 4-6   Circle of Willis.

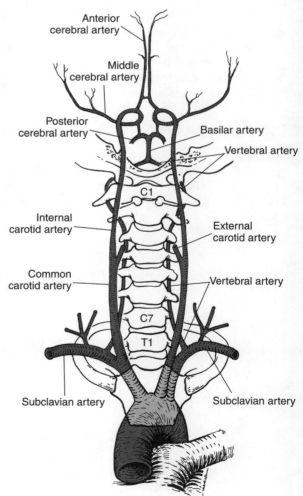

Figure 4-7   Blood supply to the brain. (**A,** From Osborn AG: *Introduction to cerebral angiography,* Hagerstown, 1980, Harper & Row.)

A

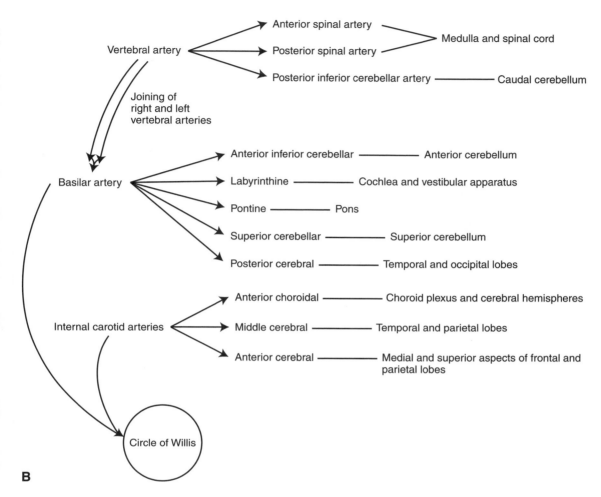

Figure 4-7—cont'd   Blood supply to the brain.

- Damage to the anterior cerebral artery leads to paralysis and loss of sensation of the contralateral leg.
- Damage to the posterior cerebral artery leads to contralateral homonymous hemianopia.
- Damage to the vertebrobasilar artery results in double vision, facial numbness and weakness, vertigo, dysphagia, dysarthria, ataxia, and motor and sensory loss in both arms and legs.
- Ischemic stroke or transient ischemic attacks cause loss of function in the affected artery of the brain.

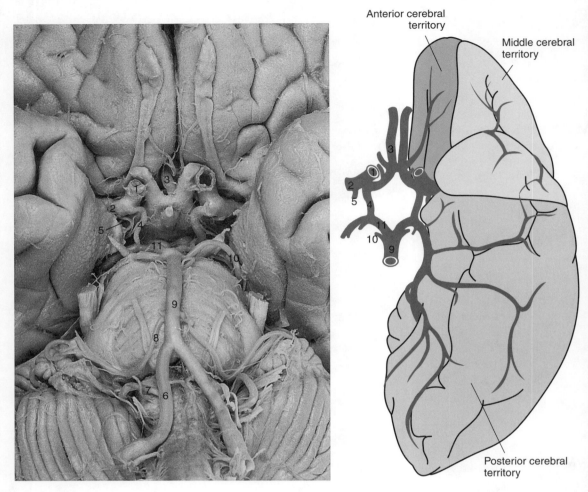

Figure 4-8   Areas supplied by anterior, middle, and posterior cerebral arteries. (Photo from Nolte J, Angevine JB Jr: *The human brain in photographs and diagrams,* ed 2, St Louis, 2000, Mosby. Illustration modified from Mettler FA: *Neuroanatomy,* ed 2, St Louis, 1948, Mosby.)

Review Questions

MENINGES

I. Fill in the Blanks

1. The brain tissue is protected by the _____ .

2. The brain is further protected by three envelopes of membranous layers: _____ _____ , _____ , and _____ .

3. The outermost covering is the _____ .

4. The middle covering is the _____ .

5. The third and the innermost layer is the very thin, delicate, and capillary-rich _____ _____ .

6. The _____ and _____ nerves supply the dura mater.

7. _____ components of all cranial nerves innervate the meninges.

8. The _____ space is filled with cerebrospinal fluid and acts as a shock absorber.

9. _____ _____ help anchor the brain to prevent it from excessive movement.

10. The _____ holds the brain tissue together and prevents it from separating.

11. All the meninges pass through the _____ _____ to enclose the spinal cord.

12. The trigeminal nerves C-1 to C-3 are the principal sensory nerves to the _____ _____ .

13. The _____ space lies between the inner bone surface and the dura mater.

14. Between the dura mater and the underlying pia mater is a narrow underlying _____ _____ .

15. The _____ space, i.e., the space between the arachnoid membrane and the pia mater, is filled with CSF.

16. CSF is secreted by the _____ plexus.

17. _____ _____ absorbs shock waves to the head.

18. Cerebral arteries and veins are situated in the _____ space.

II. Multiple Choice

1. Which of the meningeal layers is intimately attached to the surface of the brain?
   a. pia mater
   b. dura mater
   c. neither of the above

2. The meningeal layer that closely follows the contours of the brain is the _____
   _____ .
   a. dura mater
   b. pia mater
   c. arachnoid membrane

3. The meningeal layers that closely follow the contours of the cranium are the _____
   _____ .
   a. dura mater and arachnoid membrane
   b. pia mater and arachnoid membrane
   c. neither of the above

4. Dural folds lying between the cerebral hemispheres are called _____ .
   a. tentorium cerebelli
   b. falx cerebelli
   c. none of the above

5. Arachnoid trabeculations extending from the _____ help anchor the brain during shock waves.
   a. pia mater
   b. dura mater
   c. arachnoid membrane

6. Cerebral arteries and veins are situated in the _____ space.
   a. epidural
   b. subdural
   c. subarachnoid

III. True or False

1. Dura mater holds the inner brain tissues together.
2. Portions of the dura mater between two the cerebellar hemispheres are called the falx cerebri.
3. Portions of the dura mater between the two cerebral hemispheres are called the falx cerebelli.

4. Portions of the dura mater lying between the cerebellum and the occipital lobes are called the tentorium cerebri.
5. The spinal cord is surrounded by meninges that pass through the foramen magnum at the base of the skull.
6. Meningitis is infection in the meninges.
7. There is almost no space between the pia mater and the brain.

VENTRICLES AND THE CEREBROSPINAL FLUID

I. Fill in the Blanks

1. _____ is a clear fluid filling the entire subarachnoid space that acts as a liquid cushion around the brain, absorbing shocks and blows.

2. CSF is produced in the _____ _____ of each ventricle.

3. CSF flows to the third ventricle via the _____ .

4. CSF flows into the fourth ventricle via the _____ .

5. CSF leaves from three openings in the fourth ventricle and completely fills the _____ _____ around the brain and spinal cord.

6. Dural venous blood carries the excess CSF away from the subarachnoid space via the _____ granulations.

7. CSF is constantly produced at the rate of _____ ml/hour.

8. _____ is the clinical procedure where the spinal cord is punctured at a point to draw CSF for analysis.

9. Increase in _____ pressure is noticed in many pathological conditions (e.g., tumors).

10. Caused by increased intracranial pressure, _____ is noticed in the optic disc of the retina.

11. Choroid plexus (formed by pia mater) secretes _____ .

12. _____ is caused by blockage in the ventricular system.

13. _____ is one of the causes of increased intracranial pressure.

14. A decrease in intracranial pressure may cause _____ and herniation of brain tissues.

15. _____ fluid is found within the ventricular system.

16. The _____ ventricles are located within the cerebral hemispheres.

II. Multiple Choice

1. The _____ ventricle is located between the thalamus of each hemisphere.
   a. third
   b. fourth
   c. lateral

2. The _____ ventricle is located within the brainstem.
   a. third
   b. fourth

3. The _____ _____ creates CSF.
   a. choroid plexus
   b. plexiform nuclei

4. The _____ ventricle is connected to the lateral ventricle by the interventricular foramen of Monroe.
   a. third
   b. fourth
   c. neither of the above

5. The cerebral aqueduct interconnects the _____ and fourth ventricles.
   a. lateral
   b. third
   c. neither of the above

6. After exiting the fourth ventricle, CSF is located within the _____ space.
   a. subarachnoid
   b. subdural
   c. epidural

7. _____, located in the superior sagittal sinus, reabsorb CSF and move it to the systemic circulation.
   a. Arachnoid villi
   b. Dural villi
   c. Neither of the above

8. The _____ ventricle/s protect/s all lobes of the brain.
   a. Lateral
   b. Third
   c. Fourth

9. CSF is located between the _____ and _____ .
   a. arachnoid membrane; pia mater
   b. dura mater; arachnoid membrane
   c. skull; dura mater

10. _____ are cavities around which different regions of the CNS are formed.
    a. Ventricles
    b. Columns
    c. Neither of the above

BLOOD SUPPLY TO THE BRAIN

I. Fill in the Blanks

1. The vertebral and internal carotid arteries together make up the _____ artery.

2. The vertebral artery enters the skull through the _____ .

3. The _____ supplies most of the lateral surface of the hemisphere.

4. The _____ supplies the medial surface of the hemisphere.

5. Arteries arising from the _____ are called "arteries of the stroke."

6. The anastomotic ring formed between the vertebral and internal carotid arteries is called the _____ and is a frequent site for aneurysms.

7. If one path is blocked in the circle of Willis, _____ circulation becomes available.

8. Veins supplying the brain drain into the _____ .

9. Cells of the cerebral cortex are highly sensitive and they die quickly if deprived of _____ supply.

10. Epidural hematoma results from _____ .

11. Venous rupture leads to _____ hematoma.

12. _____ and _____ arteries supply blood to the brain.

II. Matching

Match the following types of strokes to the clinical conditions.

Strokes	Clinical conditions
1. Middle cerebral artery	a. cerebellar infarction with vertigo and ipsilateral cerebellar ataxia
2. Posterior cerebral artery	b. diplopia, ataxia, facial weakness
3. Basilar artery	c. contralateral homonymous hemianospia
4. Posterior inferior cerebellar artery	d. contralateral hemiparesis

III. Multiple Choice

1. The _____ cerebral artery supplies blood to the medial surface of the brain.
   a. middle
   b. anterior
   c. posterior

2. The _____ cerebral artery supplies occipital and inferior temporal lobes.
   a. middle
   b. posterior
   c. anterior

3. A physical barrier limiting diffusion of macromolecules from the blood to the extracellular

   spaces of the central nervous system is called _____ .
   a. blood-brain barrier
   b. artery barrier
   c. venous barrier

4. Two major arteries that supply blood to the brain are the vertebral and _____
   arteries.
   a. carotid
   b. basilar
   c. spinal

5. Arteries that comprise the circle of Willis are the _____ .
   a. posterior cerebral, middle cerebral, and anterior cerebral arteries
   b. posterior cerebral, posterior communicating, middle cerebral, carotid, anterior cerebral,
      and anterior communicating arteries
   c. basilar and external carotid arteries

6. The _____ cerebral artery supplies blood to the temporal lobe of the
   brain.
   a. middle
   b. anterior
   c. posterior

7. The _____ cerebral artery supplies blood to the lateral surface of the
   brain.
   a. middle
   b. anterior
   c. posterior

8. In case of _____ hemorrhage, the bleeding usually occurs from the berry
   aneurysm located near the circle of Willis.
   a. subarachnoid
   b. intracerebral
   c. subdural

9. _____ hemorrhage usually occurs in the presence of arterial hypertension,
   causing focal neurological deficits.
   a. Subarachnoid
   b. Intracerebral
   c. Subdural

10. Bleeding into the ventricular system usually leads to death within a couple of hours after

    _____ .
    a. confusion
    b. seizures
    c. coma

11. Bleeding in the area of the _____ causes massive neurological deficits
    (cranial nerve palsies, cerebellar signs, and quadriplegia), and obstructive hydrocephalus.
    a. spinal cord
    b. pons
    c. cerebellum

Answers to Review Questions

MENINGES

I. Fill in the Blanks

1. meninges

2. dura mater; arachnoid membrane; pia mater

3. dura mater

4. arachnoid membrane

5. pia mater

6. trigeminal; cervical

7. Sensory

8. subarachnoid

9. Arachnoid trabeculations

10. pia mater

11. foramen magnum

12. dura mater

13. epidural

14. arachnoid membrane

15. subarachnoid

16. choroid

17. Cerebrospinal fluid

18. subarachnoid

II. Multiple Choice

1. a   2. b   3. a   4. b   5. c   6. c

III. True or False

1. False   2. False   3. False   4. False   5. True   6. True   7. True

VENTRICLES AND THE CEREBROSPINAL FLUID

I. Fill in the Blanks

1. CSF

2. choroid plexus

3. foramen of Monroe

4. aqueduct of Sylvius

5. subarachnoid space

6. arachnoid

7. 30

8. Spinal tap

9. intracranial

10. papilledema

11. CSF

12. Hydrocephalus

13. Hydrocephalus

14. headaches

15. Cerebrospinal

16. lateral

II. Multiple Choice

1. a   3. a   5. b   7. a   9. a
2. b   4. a   6. a   8. a   10. a

BLOOD SUPPLY TO THE BRAIN
I. Fill in the Blanks

1. basilar

2. foramen magnum

3. middle cerebral artery

4. anterior cerebral artery

5. middle cerebral artery

6. circle of Willis

7. collateral

8. venous sinuses in the dura mater

9. blood

10. arterial rupture

11. subdural

12. Internal carotid; vertebral

II. Matching
1. d   2. c   3. b   4. a

III. Multiple Choice
1. b	4. a	7. a	10. c
2. b	5. b	8. a	11. b
3. a	6. a	9. b	

Cranial Nerves

The cranial nerves are named so because they originate from the hemispheric level and from the brainstem (midbrain, pons, and medulla oblongata) (Figure 5-1). Cranial nerves, along with spinal nerves, are a part of the peripheral nervous system. There are 12 pairs of cranial nerves, each of which serves specific functions. These nerves are numbered from one to twelve, usually denoted by roman numerals (I to XII).

It is important to know the location of the cranial nerves because lesions can be identified based on the signs that develop. The first two cranial nerves lie anterior to the brainstem and close to the cerebral hemisphere. The midbrain contains the nuclei of the third and fourth cranial

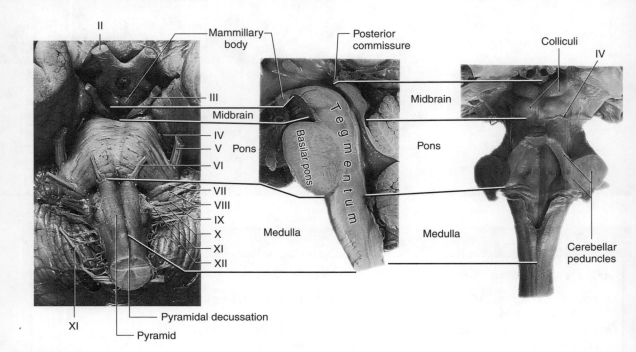

Figure 5-1   Origin of cranial nerves. (From Haines DE: *Fundamental neuroscience,* ed 2, Philadelphia, 2002, Churchill Livingstone.)

nerves. The pons contains the nuclei of the fifth, sixth, seventh, and eighth cranial nerves. The medulla oblongata is the origin of cranial nerves nine, ten, eleven, and twelve.

Based on their functions, cranial nerves serve motor, sensory, or both functions. In addition, they also carry parasympathetic fibers. Three cranial nerves (olfactory, optic, and vestibuloacoustic) serve sensory functions and five cranial nerves (oculomotor, trochlear, abducens, glossopharyngeal, and hypoglossal) have motor functions. Four cranial nerves (trigeminal, facial, glossopharyngeal, and vagus) are mixed (sensory and motor). Four cranial nerves (oculomotor, facial, glossopharyngeal, and vagus) carry parasympathetic (autonomic) fibers.

CRANIAL NERVES AND THEIR FUNCTIONS

Understanding cranial nerves and their functions is extremely important to the speech-language pathologist.

The first cranial nerve (I) is called the olfactory nerve and is related to the sense of smell. It supplies the olfactory mucosal membrane of the nose and sensory cells in the nasal cavities related to smell. It is seen in the anterolateral surface of the brainstem and at the level of the cerebrum.

The second cranial nerve (II) is called the optic nerve and it supplies the retina. This is important for communicating visual information to the brain.

The third cranial nerve (III) is called the oculomotor nerve because it helps with motor movements of the eyelids and eyeballs. Five extrinsic eye muscles are supplied by this nerve.

The fourth cranial nerve (IV) is the trochlear nerve that innervates one extraocular muscle, which is responsible for inferolateral movements of the eyes.

The fifth cranial nerve (V), the trigeminal nerve, has both sensory and motor roots. The sensory root supplies the head and face, whereas the motor root supplies the muscles of mastication. The sensory part is responsible for cutaneous (touch, temperature, and pain) and proprioceptive sensations from the face, head, and neck. The trigeminal nerve has three sensory branches: (1) ophthalmic, (2) maxillary, and (3) mandibular (Figure 5-2). The ophthalmic branch carries sensations of touch, pain, temperature, and proprioception from the skin of the forehead, anterior scalp, vertex, eyeball, upper eyelids, cornea, anterior and lateral surfaces of the nose, cornea, conjunctiva, and frontal and nasal sinuses. The maxillary branch carries sensation from the posterior surfaces of the nose, lower eyelids, upper cheeks, and upper lips. The mandibular branch carries sensations from the lower gum, mouth, and sides of the scalp. The motor part controls the muscles of mastication, which includes "TIME"—T: temporalis; I: internal pterygoid; M: masseter; and E: external pterygoid. The motor part also supplies the tensor veli palatini, a muscle of the soft palate, and the tensor tympani, a muscle of the middle ear.

The sixth cranial nerve (VI) is the abducens nerve, which supplies one extraocular muscle that helps in lateral movements of the eyes.

The seventh cranial nerve (VII), the facial nerve, mainly supplies the muscles of the face with its motor branch. The sensory branch supplies the anterior two thirds of the tongue for taste sensations and mediates sensation from the ear canal and behind the auricle. The parasympathetic fibers, a part of the autonomic nervous system, help in vasodilation and in secretion by the salivary glands (sublingual and submaxillary). Functions of this nerve are related to the secretion of tears and saliva, taste, and facial expressions.

The eighth cranial nerve (VIII) is called the vestibuloacoustic nerve, and it divides into two branches to supply the cochlear and vestibular structures. The cochlear nerve supplies the organ of Corti, which helps in hearing. The vestibular nerve supplies the semicircular canals, utricle, and saccule, which help maintain balance.

The ninth cranial nerve (IX) is the glossopharyngeal nerve and has sensory as well as motor fibers. The sensory fibers are responsible for pain, touch, and temperature sensations from the pharynx, fauces, and palatine tonsils. It also provides taste sensation to the posterior one third of the tongue. The motor fibers supply the muscles of the pharynx. It helps in swallowing.

The tenth cranial nerve (X) is the vagus nerve and it innervates the neck, thorax, and abdomen. This is the longest cranial nerve in the system and is also called the "wandering nerve." This nerve contains motor, sensory, and autonomic fibers. This nerve divides into three main branches to supply various structures of the body. The jugular branch supplies the larynx, pharynx, and superior cardiac areas. The thoracic branch supplies the inferior cardiac, bronchial, and esophageal areas. The abdominal branch supplies the gastric, celiac (abdominal), and hepatic areas. It is involved in phonation, swallowing, and regulation of cardiac, pulmonary, and gastrointestinal activities.

The eleventh cranial nerve (XI) is the accessory nerve; it supplies two neck muscles, the sternocleidomastoid and trapezius, that are important in maintaining posture of the head. It also helps during swallowing movements.

The twelfth cranial nerve (XII) is the hypoglossal nerve. This motor nerve supplies all muscles of the tongue except the glossopalatine muscle. This helps in speech and swallowing activities.

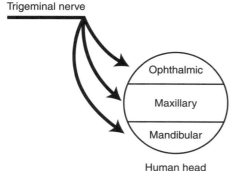

Figure 5-2   Branches of the trigeminal nerve.

EXAMINATION OF CRANIAL NERVES

To understand communication and hearing disorders, it is important to perform a systematic examination of the specific cranial nerves. These nerves must be examined to understand the structural and functional integrity of the brainstem and other related areas.

The olfactory (I) cranial nerve is tested by asking the patient to smell aromatic substances, such as cloves, cinnamon, or coffee. The patient is asked to smell the given substance placed under one nostril while occluding the other one. Different aromatic substances are tried.

The optic (II) nerve is usually tested to determine visual acuity, visual fields, and visual perception of colors. The retina of the eye is also examined.

The oculomotor (III), trochlear (IV), and abducens (VI) nerves are tested by finding out the movements of the extraocular muscles of both eyes. Movements of the eyes toward the right, left, superior, and inferior directions are tested along with elevation, depression, adduction, and abduction of eyeballs. Constriction of pupils and visual accommodation are tested to examine the parasympathetic fibers of the oculomotor nerve. Symmetry of eye movements and nystagmus are also noted while testing.

The trigeminal (V) nerve is tested for both motor and sensory functions. The sensory branch of the trigeminal nerve spreads itself in ophthalmic, mandibular, and maxillary areas of the face. The trigeminal nerve is tested by stimulating the various areas with a cotton ball. Blink reflex is also tested. The motor aspect of the nerve is examined by assessing the extent of jaw-jerk reflex, jaw-opening, jaw-closing, and rotary and vertical movements of the jaw. Jaw functions are also tested using non-vegetative activities like speech, and jaw movements during articulation of various speech sounds are noted.

The facial (VII) nerve is tested by asking the patient to smile, pucker lips, raise eyebrows, and taste different foods placed on the anterior part of the tongue.

The vestibuloacoustic (VIII) nerve is tested for hearing and balance disorders.

The glossopharyngeal (IX) nerve is tested by eliciting the gag reflex.

The vagus (X) nerve is tested by asking the patient to phonate and swallow.

The accessory (XI) nerve is tested by asking the patient to shrug the shoulders and turn the head.

The hypoglossal (XII) nerve is tested by asking the patient to perform various movements with the tongue and articulate various lingual sounds (/l/, /t/, /k/, etc.).

CLINICAL NOTES

Lesions of cranial nerves produce many and varied signs and symptoms. The knowledge of pathological conditions of cranial nerves is extremely important in the field of communication disorders. Some notes regarding specific clinical conditions are as follows:

- Damage to the seventh cranial nerve results in paralysis of the stapedius muscle in the middle ear, producing hyperacusis, in which normal sounds are perceived as louder.
- Disorders related to ocular muscles are caused by neurotransmission disorders, e.g., myasthenia gravis. Eye movement disorders also result form cortical and brainstem strokes.
- A dysfunction of any cranial nerve may be seen after closed brain injury, which may cause a nerve to be contused, lacerated, stretched, or sheared.
- If a lesion of the tenth cranial nerve is bilateral, both vocal folds will be paralyzed in the paramedian position. On respiration, inspiratory stridor will occur, and coup de glotte will be weak.
- In unilateral damage, the tongue will appear curved on protrusion. It will be weak on the side of the lesion and will deviate toward that side on protrusion. Bilateral weakness, atrophy, and fasciculations are seen during bilateral damage of the nerve. This would naturally cause dysarthria and swallowing problems (difficulty in chewing and bolus manipulation). See Table 5-1 for a more comprehensive view of cranial nerve pathologies.

TABLE 5-1	Cranial Nerve Pathologies

Cranial nerves	**Pathologies**
I. Olfactory nerve	Anosmia, hyposmia, hyperosmia
II. Optic	Visual field defects like bitemporal hemianopsia, homonymous hemianopsia, scotoma, macular sparing, etc.
III. Oculomotor	Ptosis, dilation of pupil, ophthalmoplegia, strabismus
IV. Trochlear	Upward medial gaze, diplopia
V. Trigeminal	Loss of sneezing, blinking, and corneal reflexes, trigeminal neuralgia, paralysis/paresis of muscles of mastication, jaw jerk reflex, atrophy of masticatory muscles, articulatory problems
VI. Abducens	Medial strabismus, diplopia, abnormal gaze control
VII. Facial	Facial palsy, Bell's palsy, excessive secretion from glands, loss of nasolabial folds, loss of taste to anterior two-third of the tongue and palate, inability to close eyes or raise brows, hyperacusia due to paralysis of the stapedius muscle
VIII. Vestibulocochlear	Disturbances in hearing and equilibrium, vertigo, nystagmus
IX. Glossopharyngeal	Loss of taste sensation from the posterior third of the tongue, excessive oral secretion, loss of gag reflex, paralysis of pharyngeal muscles, swallowing problems, glossopharyngeal neuralgia
X. Vagus	Loss of survival reflexes (e.g., cough, gag, swallow, etc.), paralysis of soft palate, larynx, and pharynx, dysphagia, voice disorders, loss of taste sensation from pharyngeal and epiglottic areas, anesthesia of larynx, pharynx, and associated structures
XI. Accessory	Inability to control head and shoulder movements
XII. Hypoglossal	Paralysis of tongue, atrophy and fasciculations of tongue muscles, dysarthria, dysphagia

You will be able to learn about the neuropathology of cranial nerves by answering the following questions.

Review Questions

I. Multiple Choice

1. Which cranial nerve is damaged to cause hearing loss, vertigo, nystagmus, and disequilibrium?
   a. X
   b. VII
   c. VIII
   d. XII

2. Which condition results if the second cranial nerve is damaged?
   a. visual field deficits
   b. blindness
   c. both of the above
   d. none of the above

3. Which of the following is not true about fifth cranial nerve damage?
   a. It is concerned with loss of taste.
   b. It is concerned with loss of pain and temperature.
   c. It is concerned with loss of pressure and touch sensations.
   d. It is concerned with loss of ability to masticate.

4. Which of the following cranial nerves produces pain in the facial areas after damage resulting from an unknown cause?
   a. VII
   b. IX
   c. V
   d. XI

5. Damage to the _____ cranial nerve results in upper and lower facial weakness, loss of taste, dry mouth (xerostomia), and dysarthria.
   a. tenth
   b. fifth
   c. seventh
   d. none of the above

6. Damage to the _____ cranial nerve is likely to cause _____

   _____ .
   a. third; hearing loss
   b. first; anosmia
   c. eighth; tongue paralysis
   d. twelfth; laryngeal paralysis

7. An acoustic neuroma (also called neurolemma or schwannoma) is a benign tissue growth that arises on the _____ cranial nerve and leads to hearing loss in one ear accompanied by tinnitus.
   a. sixth
   b. eighth
   c. ninth
   d. eleventh

8. A unilateral lesion in the cortex produces a contralateral paralysis of the lower face. This is caused by damage to the _____ cranial nerve.
   a. seventh
   b. eighth
   c. fifth
   d. none of the above

9. Lesions that involve the facial nerve disable dampening of sound reflexively, resulting in _____ .
   a. hypoacusis
   b. hyperacusis
   c. neither of the above.

10. Idiopathic inflammation, viral infection, or vascular compression of cranial nerve VII leads to _____ .
    a. disequilibrium
    b. loss of smell
    c. Bell's palsy
    d. vision disorders

11. Trigeminal neuralgia or tic douloureux, which is caused by a _____ nerve lesion, is characterized by intermittent, shooting pain in the face.
    a. seventh
    b. eighth
    c. fifth
    d. tenth

12. When an abnormal arterial loop irritates the _____ nerve, hemifacial spasm takes place, characterized by intermittent or continuous twitching of one side of the face.
    a. glossopharyngeal
    b. facial
    c. trigeminal
    d. vagus

13. _____ neuralgia, although not as common as trigeminal neuralgia, is characterized by shooting pain in the throat, tonsil region, and base of the tongue on one side. The pain may be spontaneous and is triggered by swallowing.
    a. Facial
    b. Trigeminal
    c. Hypoglossal
    d. None of the above

14. Diplopia may be caused by damage to cranial nerves, ——————————— , ——————————— , and ——————————— .
    a. III; IV; V
    b. III; IV; VII
    c. III; IV; IX
    d. III; IV; VI

15. Cranial nerve ——————————— is frequently disrupted after traumatic brain injury.
    a. IX
    b. I
    c. X
    d. XII

16. Damage to the ——————————— cranial nerve results in dysphagia, dysarthria, loss of taste, anesthesia of the pharynx, and dryness of mouth.
    a. tenth
    b. twelfth
    c. ninth
    d. eighth

17. Bitemporal hemianopsia (tunnel vision) may be caused by lesions in the optic chiasm (crossing over of optic fibers before entering the thalamus and cortex). Postchiasmatic lesions are associated with homonymous hemianopsia or quadranopsia, depending on the location of the lesion. These disorders are caused by damage to cranial nerve ——————————— .
    a. III
    b. II
    c. IV
    d. VI

18. Trauma to the petrous bone in the skull will result in damage to cranial nerves ——————— ——————————— and VIII, leading to facial weakness, loss of taste sensation in the anterior two-thirds of the tongue, and deafness.
    a. II
    b. VII
    c. IX
    d. X

19. Weak gag reflex and reduced phonation are caused by ——————————— cranial nerve damage.
    a. tenth
    b. twelfth
    c. seventh
    d. ninth

20. Loss of tactile sensations over mouth, tongue, and hard palate is caused by damage to the

    _____ division of the _____ cranial nerve.
    a. motor; fifth
    b. sensory; seventh
    c. sensory; tenth
    d. sensory; fifth

21. Vocal cords are paralyzed in the paramedian position when there is a unilateral lesion in

    the recurrent laryngeal nerve, a division of cranial nerve _____ . The
    consequences are breathy voice, diphthongia, and hoarseness.
    a. IX
    b. XI
    c. VII
    d. X

22. Unilateral damage to cranial nerve _____ leads to atrophy and fascicu-
    lations of the tongue on the side of the lesion.
    a. V
    b. VII
    c. XII
    d. X

23. Nasal regurgitation (loss of food or fluid through the nose) is a result of a _____

    _____ nerve lesion; other signs are soft palate paralysis, pharyngeal
    paralysis, and dysphagia.
    a. fifth
    b. tenth
    c. seventh
    d. twelfth

24. Resonance and articulation disorders are caused by damage to cranial nerve _____

    _____ .
    a. VIII
    b. IX
    c. VI
    d. V

25. Postural problems and general tonicity of the neck regions take place when cranial nerve

    _____ is damaged. This indirectly affects resonation in speech.
    a. X
    b. IX
    c. XII
    d. XI

26. Jaw jerk reflex will be absent because of damage to cranial nerve _____ .
    a. VII
    b. XII
    c. XI
    d. none of the above

27. Damage to the nucleus ambiguous, one of the nuclei of the _____ cranial nerve, results in ipsilateral paresis/paralysis of the pharynx and soft palate, leading to a swallowing disorder.
    a. seventh
    b. ninth
    c. tenth
    d. eleventh

28. Damage to the sensory part of cranial nerve _____ leads to anesthesia of the larynx, pharynx, and loss of taste sensation from pharyngeal and epiglottic areas.
    a. VII
    b. IX
    c. X
    d. none of the above

II. Fill in the Blanks

1. There are _____ pairs of cranial nerves.

2. They are called cranial nerves because _____ .

3. The cranial nerves have _____ , _____ , _____ , and _____ types of fibers.

4. Cranial nerve I is _____ in nature.

5. The blink reflex is related to cranial nerve _____ .

6. The _____ cranial nerve helps elevate our eyelids.

7. The mandibular branch belongs to cranial nerve _____ .

8. If cranial nerve _____ is damaged, the jaw-jerk reflex will be affected.

9. The vestibuloocular reflex is linked to the _____ cranial nerve.

10. Cranial nerve _____ contributes to taste functions in the anterior two thirds of the tongue.

11. The gag reflex will be abnormal because of damage to cranial nerves _____ and _____ .

12. The hypoglossal nerve is _____ in nature.

13. The nuclei of cranial nerves ——————————— , ——————————— , ——————————— , and ——————————— exist in the medulla.

14. Lingual paralysis is caused by damage to cranial nerve ——————————— .

15. Delayed swallow response, aspiration, and absence of gag reflex are characteristics of ——————————— cranial nerve damage.

16. Muscular atrophy of the tongue is noted when there has been lower motor neuron damage of cranial nerve ——————————— .

17. The ——————————— cranial nerve innervates the muscles of mastication.

18. The ——————————— cranial nerve supplies one of the muscles of the middle ear, called the tensor tympani.

19. Cranial nerve ——————————— mediates auditory and vestibular sensations.

20. Cranial nerve ——————————— supplies the intrinsic laryngeal muscles.

III. Matching

Match the disorders with their respective cranial nerves.

1. Anosmia	XII
2. Hoarseness of voice	VII
3. Weakness of tongue	II
4. Facial palsy	IX
5. Hemianopsia	V
6. Facial pain	III
7. Vertigo and tinnitus	X
8. Soft palate palsy	VIII
9. Ophthalmoplegia	I

IV. Fill in the Blanks

Give a brief description of what each cranial nerve does. These cranial nerves are important in understanding communication disorders.

1. Cranial nerve V: ——————————————————————————

2. Cranial nerve VII ——————————————————————————

3. Cranial nerve VIII ——————————————————————————

4. Cranial nerve IX ——————————————————————————

5. Cranial nerve X ——————————————————————————

6. Cranial nerve XI _____

7. Cranial nerve XII _____

V. Fill in the Blanks

Name the cranial nerves that are important for the following functions.

1. Hearing: _____

2. Smell: _____

3. Balance: _____

4. Vision: _____

5. Taste: _____

6. Swallowing: _____

7. Eye movements: _____

8. Temperature sensations on the face: _____

9. Production of consonants: _____

10. Head positioning: _____

11. Phonation: _____

12. Production of nasal sounds: _____

Answers to Review Questions

I. Multiple Choice

1. c	5. c	9. b	13. d	17. b	21. d
2. c	6. b	10. c	14. d	18. b	22. c
3. a	7. b	11. c	15. b	19. a	23. b
4. c	8. a	12. b	16. c	20. d	24. b

II. Fill in the Blanks

1. 12

2. they exit from the level of the cranium (brainstem)

3. motor, sensorimotor, sensory, visceral

4. sensory

5. V

6. third

7. V

8. V

9. eighth

10. VII

11. IX and X

12. motor

13. IX, X, XI, XII

14. XII

15. tenth

16. XII

17. fifth

18. fifth

19. VIII

20. X

III. Matching

1. I	4. VII	7. VIII
2. X	5. II	8. IX
3. XII	6. V	9. III

IV. Fill in the Blanks

1. Cranial nerve V: Supplies skin of face; mucosa of nasal, oral, and orbital cavities; teeth; meninges; anterior two thirds of the tongue for pain, temperature, pressure, and touch sensations; external surface of the tympanic membrane; and muscles of mastication.

2. Cranial nerve VII: Supplies anterior two thirds of the tongue and palate for taste; muscles of facial expression; lacrimal gland; skin of the external ear; and salivary glands except the parotid.

3. Cranial nerve VIII: Supplies cochlea, semicircular canals, utricle, and saccule.

4. Cranial nerve IX: Supplies mucosa of upper pharynx, skin of external ear, middle ear cavity, posterior one third of the tongue for taste, pharyngeal muscles, and parotid glands.

5. Cranial nerve X: Supplies pharyngeal and laryngeal areas, epiglottis, thoracic and abdominal viscera, skin of external ear, extrinsic and intrinsic muscles of the pharynx and larynx, heart, glands, and smooth muscles.

6. Cranial nerve XI: Supplies muscles of the neck.

7. Cranial nerve XII: Supplies the intrinsic and extrinsic muscles of the tongue except the palatoglossus.

V. Fill in the Blanks

1. VIII

2. I

3. VIII

4. II

5. VII, IX

6. V, VII, IX, X, XI, XII

7. III, IV, VI

8. V

9. V, VII, IX, X, XII

10. XI

11. X

12. IX

The Central Auditory Nervous System

S ound travels from the external ear to the middle ear and then the inner ear. The external ear consists of the pinna and the external auditory canal, which serves as a resonating chamber. The middle ear is an air-filled cavity that contains tiny bones called ossicles. These ossicles, specifically, the malleus, incus, and stapes, modify the sound so it can travel via a fluid-filled structure in the inner ear called the cochlea. When cochlear fluids sense the vibrations, the sensory hair cells release a neurotransmitter that excites the auditory nerve (cranial nerve VIII). Auditory processing does not end in the ear itself. All information is delivered through the auditory nerve to the brainstem, where it travels up a complex neural pathway to its final destination, the cortex, for ultimate interpretation.

PATHWAYS FOR AUDITORY REFLEXES

When a sound is heard, auditory reflexes coordinate head and eye movements toward the sound source for the purpose of localization. The inferior colliculus projects to the superior colliculus and tectum of the midbrain, thus integrating auditory and visual systems. Another pathway starts from the superior olivary complex and projects to cranial nerves III, IV, and VI, which are responsible for eye movements. Thus ocular movements occur in response to auditory stimuli. Via another pathway, auditory nuclei connect to the vestibular nuclei in the brainstem and cerebellum.

ASCENDING AUDITORY PATHWAYS (FIGURES 6-1 THROUGH 6-3)

Auditory signals are carried from the inner ear to the brain via a pathway with many synapses. The cochlear nerve, a branch of the vestibulocochlear nerve (cranial nerve VIII) emerges from the internal acoustic meatus and continues to the junction of the medulla and pons. The afferent fibers then bifurcate, one branch ending in the dorsal cochlear nucleus (DCN) and the other branch in the ventral cochlear nucleus (VCN). These nuclei are located in the rostral end of the

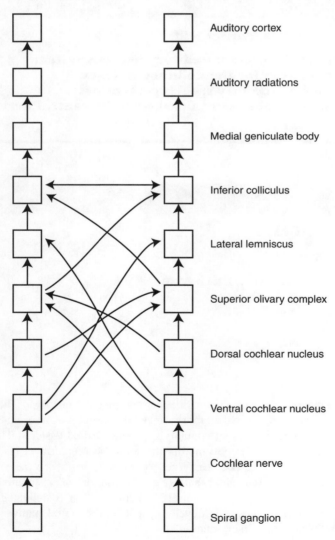

Auditory cortex

Auditory radiations

Medial geniculate body

Inferior colliculus

Lateral lemniscus

Superior olivary complex

Dorsal cochlear nucleus

Ventral cochlear nucleus

Cochlear nerve

Spiral ganglion

Figure 6-1   Auditory pathways.

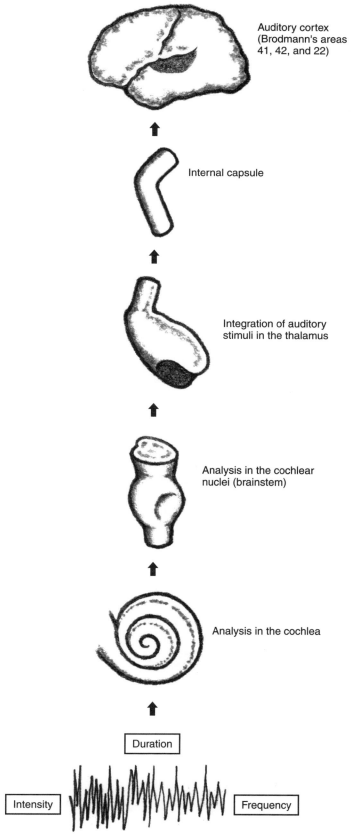

Figure 6-2 A crude model of auditory processing of speech.

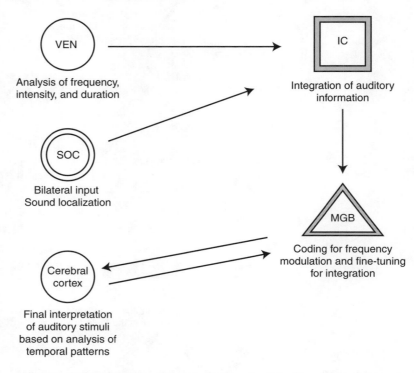

Figure 6-3   Neural encoding of acoustic stimuli in the auditory pathways.

medulla. From these nuclei the pathways (both contralateral and ipsilateral) to the cerebral cortex are characterized by one or more synaptic relays between the cochlear nuclei and specific thalamic nucleus. The auditory nerve leaves the medulla and enters the tegmentum of the pons, where the superior olivary complex (SOC) is located. There are other synaptic connections in the lateral lemniscus and the inferior colliculus of the midbrain. After leaving the midbrain, the auditory nerve enters the thalamus, which contains the medial geniculate body, a special nucleus for hearing. The last link in the auditory pathway consists of the auditory radiation, through which the medial geniculate body projects onto the primary auditory cortex of the temporal lobe (Figure 6-4).

According to tonotopic organization a single neuron in the nucleus responds best to certain sound frequencies. Fibers from the apex of the cochlea, which carries low-frequency information, end up in the superficial layers of the cochlear nucleus; fibers carrying high-frequency information from the base of the cochlea terminate in the deeper layers of the cochlear nuclei.

DESCENDING FIBERS IN THE AUDITORY PATHWAY

The function of descending auditory projections is to refine the perception of pitch and loudness through the process of inhibition. Efferent neurons conduct impulses in the reverse direction, thereby providing the feedback circuits. The descending connections consist of the corticogeniculate fibers (projection from cortical areas to the medial geniculate body); corticocollicular fibers (projection from cortex to inferior colliculus); colliculo-olivary fibers (projection from the inferior colliculus to the superior olivary complex); olivocochlear fibers (projection from superior olivary complex to the cochlear nuclei); and colliculocochleonuclear fibers (projection from inferior colliculus to the dorsal and ventral cochlear nucleus). The descending pathways are mostly ipsilateral except for the corticocollicular projection.

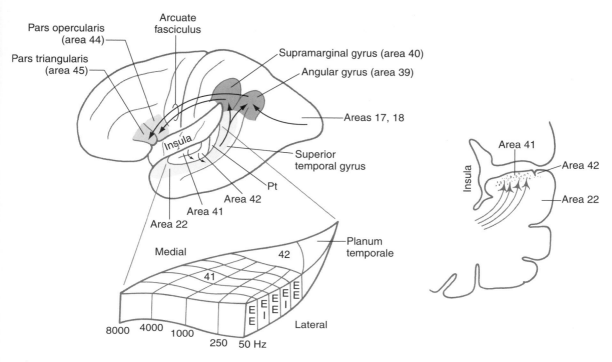

Figure 6-4 Auditory cortex. (From Haines DE: *Fundamental neuroscience,* ed 2, Philadelphia, 2002, Churchill Livingstone.)

CLINICAL NOTES

- Sensorineural deafness is caused by interruption of cochlear nerve fibers from hair cells to the brainstem nuclei.
- Acoustic neuroma is a benign tumor on the cells of the vestibular component of the vestibulo-cochlear nerve. The triad of symptoms consists of hearing loss, tinnitus, and vertigo. Vertigo is characterized by intermittent or progressive unsteadiness. The tumor sometimes occupies the cerebellopontine angle in the intracranial space.
- Disorders that can affect processing of sound through the cerebrum include degenerative diseases such as multiple sclerosis, amyotrophic lateral sclerosis, Parkinson's and Alzheimer's disease, aphasia, and anoxia.
- Central auditory processing dysfunction is caused by any lesion in the auditory pathways. The individual affected has difficulty processing or interpreting auditory information, even though peripheral hearing is normal. Any disturbance along the auditory pathway can interfere with processing the sound into meaningful information. Damage to the auditory pathway, in general, may lead to difficulties in sound localization; auditory performance, with competing acoustic signals and degraded signals; auditory discrimination; and temporal aspects of audition, including temporal resolution, temporal masking, temporal integration, and temporal ordering.

Review Questions

I. Multiple Choice

1. The function of the outer ear is _____ .
   a. transfer of sound energy to the tympanic membrane
   b. sound localization
   c. formation of neural impulse
   d. a and b

2. The _____ ear transfers the airborne sound pressure fluctuations to the cochlea.
   a. inner
   b. middle
   c. external

3. The malleus, incus, and stapes are three bones of the _____ chain that help in sound transmission from the middle ear to the inner ear.
   a. ossicular
   b. inner ear
   c. external ear

4. Two small muscles attached to the ossicles are the stapedius and _____ , which contract to protect the ear from loud damaging sounds.
   a. depressor tympani
   b. levator tympani
   c. tensor tympani

5. The inner ear is located in the petrous part of the _____ bone.
   a. frontal
   b. parietal
   c. temporal

6. The eighth cranial nerve, also called the vestibulocochlear nerve, has two branches: the _____ and the cochlear.
   a. acoustic
   b. vestibular
   c. neither of the above

7. The ventrocochlear nucleus is the place for analysis of _____ .
   a. timing
   b. intensity
   c. frequency
   d. all of the above

8. The _____ takes part in analyzing the timing and loudness of sounds.
   a. superior olivary complex
   b. ventral cochlear nucleus
   c. dorsal cochlear nucleus

9. The _____ is used for sound localization in space.
   a. inferior colliculus
   b. ventral cochlear nucleus
   c. superior olivary complex

10. Temporal sequencing is performed by the _____ .
    a. cochlear nucleus
    b. medial geniculate body
    c. cortex
    d. all the above

11. Quality of sound is interpreted in the _____ .
    a. inferior colliculus
    b. dorsal cochlear nucleus
    c. superior olivary complex

12. The frequency information present in the firing patterns of auditory nerve fibers is present

    in the _____ .
    a. pons
    b. medulla
    c. cochlear nucleus

13. The _____ is the main auditory relay center, where integration of auditory information and somesthetic input takes place.
    a. inferior colliculus
    b. medial geniculate body
    c. superior olivary complex

14. The _____ is the thalamic relay center to the temporal lobe.
    a. inferior colliculus
    b. medial geniculate body
    c. lateral geniculate body

15. The _____ is responsible for complete sound localization, discrimination, analysis of complex sounds, and selective attention to specific auditory stimuli.
    a. thalamus
    b. inferior colliculus
    c. auditory cortex

16. Hair cells in the cochlea generate action potentials, which travel to the brainstem through

    the fibers of the _____ .
    a. trigeminal/fifth cranial nerve
    b. facial/seventh cranial nerve
    c. vestibuloacoustic nerve/eighth cranial nerve

17. The central auditory pathway extends from the cochlear nucleus complex to the primary auditory cortex or the _____ .
    a. inferior temporal gyrus
    b. Heschl's gyrus
    c. Wernicke's area

18. The superior olivary complex is a collection of nuclei situated in the _____ .
    a. medulla
    b. pons
    c. midbrain

19. The inferior colliculus is situated in the _____ .
    a. medulla
    b. pons
    c. midbrain

20. The superior olivary complex integrates time and intensity differences received from both ears and thus contributes to _____ localization of the sound.
    a. temporal
    b. spatial
    c. neither of the above

21. The auditory pathways are unique because of their multiple synaptic relays at various levels between the cochlear nuclei and the _____ .
    a. midbrain
    b. pons
    c. thalamus

22. The primary auditory cortex is also known as Brodmann's areas _____ .
    a. 41 and 42
    b. 22 and 45
    c. 21 and 44

23. The secondary auditory area is also called _____ area.
    a. Heschl's
    b. Wernicke's
    c. supramarginal

24. According to the tonotopic organization of the primary auditory cortex, higher frequency fibers terminate in the posteromedial region of the Heschl's gyrus, whereas low-frequency fibers terminate in the _____ region.
    a. anterolateral
    b. lateral
    c. medial

25. Heschl's gyrus is absolutely essential for frequency discrimination based on _____

    _____ patterns of auditory events.
    a. intensity
    b. timing
    c. none of the above

26. Bilateral representation at the cortex is the result of _____ .
    a. structural properties of the cochlea
    b. descending cortical projections
    c. multiple crossings of auditory information through ascending cortical projections

27. A lesion at any point along the central auditory nervous system causes a _____

    _____ hearing loss.
    a. profound
    b. mild
    c. severe

28. The interaural time and intensity differences play an important role in _____

    _____ .
    a. bilateral auditory representation
    b. sound localization
    c. auditory reflexes

29. Hearing loss associated with a brainstem lesion is called _____ deafness.
    a. peripheral
    b. central
    c. total

30. A peripheral lesion in the eighth cranial nerve with loss of hearing, such as a cerebello-
    pontine angle tumor, usually involves both cochlear and vestibular fibers, thus resulting in

    _____ .
    a. deafness, tinnitus, and vertigo
    b. conductive deafness
    c. mixed deafness

31. _____ is responsible for recognition, associations, and recall of auditory
    signals.
    a. Heschl's gyrus
    b. Wernicke's area
    c. Supramarginal gyrus

32. _____ mechanisms make up the auditory pathways.
    a. Peripheral hearing
    b. Neural encoding
    c. Speech perception

33. The _____ is important for the timing and duration of sound, whereas the _____ interprets the quality of the sound.
    a. ventral cochlear nucleus; dorsal cochlear nucleus
    b. dorsal cochlear nucleus; ventral cochlear nucleus
    c. basilar membrane; ventral cochlear nucleus

34. Efferent fibers from the superior olivary complex to the cochlea, the olivocochlear bundle, _____ .
    a. modulate the sensitivity of the cochlear organ
    b. enhance bilateral representation in the cortex
    c. aid in timing analysis in the cochlea

35. The _____ relays information about the frequency, intensity, and phase of a sound stimulus.
    a. cochlea
    b. middle ear
    c. auditory nerve

36. The _____ is sensitive to intensity and durational aspects of sound and is involved in acoustic startle reflex along with inferior colliculus.
    a. lateral lemniscus
    b. superior olivary complex
    c. dorsal cochlear nucleus

Answers to Review Questions

I. Multiple Choice

1. d	6. b	11. b	16. c	21. c	26. c	31. b	36. a
2. b	7. d	12. c	17. b	22. a	27. b	32. b	
3. a	8. b	13. a	18. c	23. b	28. b	33. b	
4. c	9. c	14. b	19. c	24. a	29. b	34. a	
5. c	10. d	15. c	20. a	25. b	30. a	35. c	

The Neurological Bases of the Balance Mechanism

After completing this chapter, the learner will:

- Appreciate the importance of the vestibular system, its components, and the vestibular pathways.
- Be able to list the common dysfunctions of the vestibular apparatus.

THE VESTIBULAR SYSTEM

The human inner ear contains two divisions: the cochlear system (hearing) and the vestibular system (balance). The vestibular system consists of the following components:
- Peripheral vestibular receptors (semicircular canals, utricle, and saccule)
- Vestibular branch of vestibuloacoustic nerve
- Vestibular nuclei
- Projections of nuclei

The overall functions of the vestibular system are as follows:
- Maintenance of body posture
- Coordination of body, head, and eye movements
- Visual fixation

PATHWAYS FOR BALANCE

The oval window of the middle ear opens into a large central area within the inner ear called the vestibule. The vestibule houses the cochlea, semicircular canals, utricle, and saccule. The membranous labyrinth, which contains the peripheral vestibular receptors, is filled with endolymph and surrounded by perilymph. As the position of the head changes, endolymph moves and bends the sensory hair cells. As a result, nerve impulses are created that travel along the vestibular pathways to the brain. The endolymph moves under acceleration or deceleration, and these fluid movements help detect and interpret cues concerning gravity and acceleration.

The peripheral vestibular receptors provide vital information to the brain about motion and orientation in earth's gravity. The utricle and saccule help detect linear acceleration, whereas the semicircular canals deal with angular acceleration. The utricle and saccule also contain otoliths (calcium carbonate crystals), which respond to horizontal and vertical acceleration.

The auditory and vestibular systems are intimately connected because the receptors for both are located in the temporal bone. The vestibular system is also closely associated with the visual and proprioceptive systems. Constant integration of visual and proprioceptive information by the vestibular system leads to the execution of complex and coordinated acts.

Complex vestibuloanatomic relationships involve the vestibular pathways, cerebellum, brainstem, and caudate nucleus. These sense nausea, vomiting, increased heart rate and respiration, and other symptoms common to vestibular impairments.

CLINICAL NOTES

- Peripheral vestibular nystagmus results from stimulation of the peripheral vestibular apparatus and is usually accompanied by vertigo.
- Optokinetic nystagmus occurs when there is a continuous movement of the visual field past the eyes.
- Vertigo is caused by a disturbance in equilibrium, which is an illusory feeling of spinning, falling, or disorientation in space. It is an important clinical sign related to labyrinthine diseases, tumors, and Meniere's syndrome.
- Vestibular ataxia is characterized by clumsy, uncoordinated movements, vertigo, and nystagmus.
- Patients with bilateral vestibular loss experience the apparent movement of objects within the visual field during high-frequency head movements. This condition is called oscillopsia. Patients with this disorder have no vestibulo-ocular reflex so they cannot maintain gaze stabilization.
- Patients with vestibular disorders usually visit the clinic with complaints of blurred vision, poor balance, vertigo, and spatial disorientation.

Review Questions

I. Multiple Choice

1. The _____ system is used to control bodily balance, posture, and spatial orientation.
   a. auditory
   b. vestibular
   c. peripheral nervous

2. The _____ ear, which contains the vestibule, holds the vestibular system.
   a. inner
   b. middle
   c. outer

3. The sensors for the vestibular system lie inside the _____ labyrinth.
   a. bony
   b. membranous
   c. neither of the above

4. _____ is used to look at the integrity of the vestibular pathways by noting responses to sudden changes in motion.
   a. Romberg test
   b. Positional testing
   c. Caloric testing

5. _____ is the most useful diagnostic indication of pathology of the vestibular system.
   a. Nystagmus
   b. Hearing loss
   c. Tinnitus

6. The _____ function to detect angular acceleration.
   a. tricle
   b. saccule
   c. semicircular canals

7. The _____ and _____ are meant for detecting linear acceleration.
   a. utricle; semicircular canals
   b. saccule; semicircular canals
   c. utricle; saccule

8. The lateral vestibulospinal tract helps in _____ .
   a. maintaining upright posture via control over limbs
   b. maintaining normal position of head and neck
   c. mediating the vestibulo-ocular reflex

9. The medial vestibulospinal tract helps in _____ .
   a. maintaining upright posture via control over limbs
   b. maintaining normal position of head and neck
   c. mediating the vestibulo-ocular reflex

10. The ampulla, a swollen base in the semicircular canal, contains hair cells within a receptor area called the _____ .
    a. otolith
    b. crista ampullaris
    c. macula

11. A gelatinous mass called the _____ covers each ampulla and is displaced when the head rotates.
    a. macula
    b. cupula
    c. otolith

12. Sensory hair cells are clustered in the _____ region of the utricle and saccule.
    a. macular
    b. otolithic
    c. cupular

13. The _____ fibers conduct impulses to the motor neurons of the neck muscles, leading to an adjustment of tone in the neck when the head is turned to one side.
    a. vestibulospinal
    b. vestibular
    c. cerebellar

14. Vestibular fibers terminate in the vestibular nuclear complex in the _____ .
    a. pons
    b. medulla
    c. midbrain

15. The _____ nerve fibers carry information concerning body equilibrium to the vestibular nuclei in the brainstem.
    a. vestibular
    b. cochlear
    c. vestibular and cochlear

16. Vestibular nerve fibers enter the brainstem at the _____ junction and terminate in the vestibular nuclear complex.
    a. cerebellopontine
    b. pontomedullary
    c. cerebellomedullary

17. Destruction of vestibular nuclei causes _____ .
    a. tinnitus
    b. vertigo
    c. deafness

18. The _____ vestibulospinal tract (ipsilateral) acts on limb muscles especially to maintain an upright posture, and the _____ vestibulospinal tract helps maintain normal position of the head and innervates neck muscles.
    a. lateral; medial
    b. medial; lateral
    c. superior; lateral

19. Involuntary, alternating, rapid, and slow movements of the eyeballs secondary to lesions in the vestibular apparatus are called _____ .
    a. ballismus
    b. nystagmus
    c. vertigo

20. A compensatory adjustment of gaze to keep the eyes fixed on an object during head movements is the result of the _____ , which is mediated by the medial longitudinal fasciculus.
    a. righting reflex
    b. ocular reflex
    c. vestibulo-ocular reflex

21. The vestibular ganglion is located in the _____ .
    a. internal auditory meatus
    b. organ of Corti
    c. utricle

22. The vestibular nuclei are located in the _____ .
    a. medulla
    b. pons
    c. midbrain

II. Fill in the Blanks

Identify the following vestibular pathways in Figures 7-1 through 7-5.

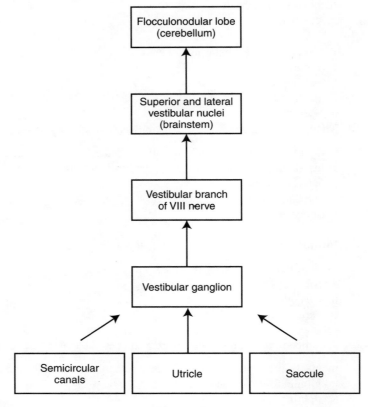

Figure 7-1

1. _____ tract

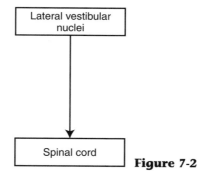

Figure 7-2

2. _____ tract

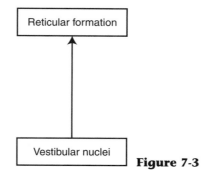

Figure 7-3

3. _____ tract

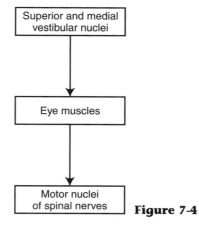

Figure 7-4

4. _____ tract

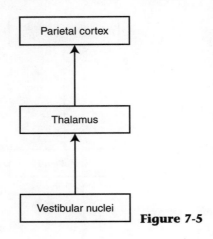

Figure 7-5

5. _____ tract

Answers to Review Questions

I. Multiple Choice

1. b	4. b	7. c	10. b	13. a	16. b	19. b	22. b
2. a	5. a	8. a	11. b	14. a	17. b	20. c	
3. b	6. c	9. b	12. a	15. a	18. a	21. c	

II. Fill in the Blanks

1. Vestibulocerebellar

2. Lateral vestibulospinal

3. Vestibuloreticular

4. Medial vestibulospinal

5. Vestibulocortical

Sensory Pathways in the Nervous System

OUTLINE

SENSORY SYSTEM

A sensory system consists of sense organs, ganglia, nuclei, and specific tracts that help carry the sensations to the cerebral cortex. The sensory system carries information from the body's sensory receptors to the central nervous system for interpretation. There are many types of sensory pathways, which are composed of specialized neurons. These neurons help transmit information to the higher cortical centers through the primary afferents, spinal cord, brainstem, and thalamus. They are arranged systemically from the first order neuron through the fourth order neuron.

PAIN AND TEMPERATURE PATHWAYS, PROPRIOCEPTION PATHWAYS, AND PRESSURE AND TOUCH PATHWAYS

The three major sensory pathways are as follows: (1) discriminative touch, (2) pain and temperature, and (3) proprioception (Figures 8-1 to 8-3). A common pathway exists for mediating discriminative touch, proprioception, and vibration. This pathway is also called the dorsal column-medial lemniscal system. It starts from the receptor areas in the muscles, tendons, joints, and skin. The nerve fibers then form the dorsal root ganglion and pass into the ipsilateral dorsal white columns of the spinal cord. From here, it goes to the medulla where the second-order neurons are found. After leaving the medulla, the fibers form a bundle called medial lemniscus, which ascends to the ventral posterolateral nucleus of the thalamus. The third-order neurons originating in the thalamus reach the postcentral gyrus in the cortex through the internal capsule.

The pathway for pain and temperature, also known as the lateral spinothalamic tract starts from the receptors on the skin. The first-order neurons form the dorsal root ganglion and enter the dorsal horn of the spinal cord through the dorsal root. Here, the second-order neurons start and they cross-over to enter into the opposite ventral white commissure. After continuing through the lateral columns, the fibers reach the ventral posterolateral nucleus of the thalamus. The third-order neurons start here and reach the postcentral gyrus of the cortex via the internal capsule.

VISUAL PATHWAY

The visual system includes the eyes and related neuronal structures of the visual pathways. The amount of space that can be seen without eye or head movements is called the visual field. At the point called the optic chiasm, optic nerve tract fibers from each side of the visual field

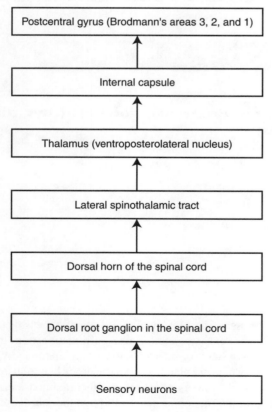

Figure 8-1 Pain and temperature pathway.

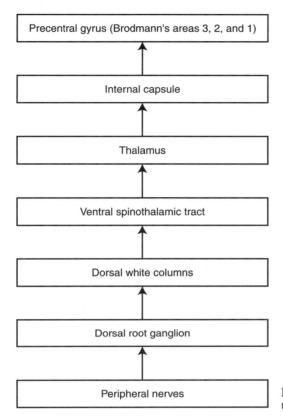

Figure 8-2   Pathway for pressure and simple touch.

decussate (cross or intersect) and then travel to the thalamus. The lateral geniculate nucleus in the thalamus projects to the primary visual cortex (also known as Brodmann's area 17) as optic radiations (Figure 8-4).

CLINICAL NOTES

- Neuralgia refers to pain in the nerves.
- Syringomyelia is a rare degenerative disease of the spinal cord that is characterized by loss of pain and temperature sensations and dissociative anesthesia.
- A damage to the sensory pathways leads to various types of sensory losses, which are expressed either contralaterally or ipsilaterally. A lesion of the lateral spinothalamic tract results in loss of pain and sensation. A lesion in the anterior spinothalamic tract results in contralateral loss of crude touch and pressure sensation. A dorsal column pathway lesion leads to proprioceptive deficits.
- Astereognosis is the loss of ability to distinguish between objects through touch and manipulation.
- The inability to distinguish two tactile points from a single one is called two-point discrimination disorder. It occurs when there is a dorsal column lesion.
- Loss of sense of vibration, loss of two-point tactile discrimination, and loss of proprioceptive sense (sensation of body in space) also characterize some sensory disorders.
- Damage to the postcentral gyrus of the parietal lobe or dorsal column pathways may produce proprioceptive deficits, loss of two-point discrimination, and loss of vibratory sense.

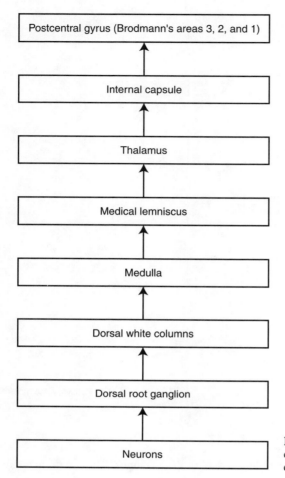

Postcentral gyrus (Brodmann's areas 3, 2, and 1)

Internal capsule

Thalamus

Medical lemniscus

Medulla

Dorsal white columns

Dorsal root ganglion

Neurons

Figure 8-3 Pathway for proprioception, discriminatory touch, and vibratory senses from the extremities and trunk.

- Damage to the spinocerebellar tract also causes proprioceptive deficits.
- Lesions in the medial longitudinal fasciculus cause impairments in oculomotor control and gaze stabilization, sometimes indicated by complaints of blurred vision.
- Blindness of one eye is caused by complete lesions of the optic nerve. This may result from nerve compression by tumors, traumatic transaction, infarction of the nerve, or demyelination.
- Bilateral hemianopia is caused by compression of the decussating fibers of the optic chiasm by a tumor.
- Homonymous hemianopia results from a lesion in the optic tract, optic radiation, or visual cortex on the opposite side. The usual causes are tumor, intracerebral hemorrhage, or cerebral infarction.
- A lesion in the anterior part of optic radiations causes a characteristic loss of vision in one quarter of the visual field.
- Lesions in the visual association cortex result in difficulty with color vision and perception of movements.
- Lesions in the temporo-occipital cortex produce dyslexia and visual agnosias.
- A lesion in the temporal lobe through which the optic radiation passes causes a visual field deficit.

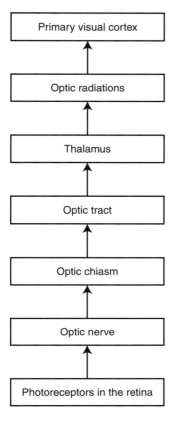

Figure 8-4   Visual pathway.

Review Questions

I. Multiple Choice

1. Pain and temperature fibers are concentrated in the lateral white columns, whereas the pressure and simple touch axons are situated in the _____ part.
    a. medial
    b. ventromedial
    c. mediolateral

2. Somatosensory pathways have a _____ organization.
    a. two-neuron
    b. three-neuron
    c. four-neuron

3. First-order somatic neurons have their cell bodies in the _____ .
    a. dorsal root ganglion
    b. dorsal horn of the spinal cord
    c. medulla

4. Second-order neurons are located in the _____ .
    a. spinal cord
    b. brainstem
    c. a and b
    d. none of the above

5. The _____ contains the third-order neurons for all types of somatic sensations.
    a. hypothalamus
    b. thalamus
    c. internal capsule

6. Third-order neurons related to somatic sensations project to the _____ area in the parietal lobe.
    a. secondary sensory
    b. primary sensory
    c. neither of the above

7. The anterior spinothalamic tract conveys _____ .
    a. unconscious proprioception
    b. diffuse touch
    c. pain

8. Conditions that affect one's ability to process fine discriminative touch and related information include _____ .
   a. inflammation of the dorsal root ganglion
   b. vascular infarcts in the cord
   c. neoplasms in the cord
   d. all of the above

9. The _____ is responsible for a finer analysis of sensation and determines its quality and source.
   a. primary sensory cortex
   b. secondary sensory cortex
   c. a and b
   d. none of the above

10. The anterior or ventral spinothalamic tract carries sensory information concerning _____ .
   a. light touch
   b. pressure
   c. a and b
   d. none of the above

11. The spinocerebellar pathway is one of the _____ pathways.
   a. sensory
   b. motor
   c. proprioceptive

12. _____ pathways help mediate conscious proprioception, two-point discrimination, and form perception.
   a. Anterior spinocerebral
   b. Medial cerebellar
   c. Dorsal column

13. There is a crossing of optic nerve fibers at the _____ .
   a. optic radiation
   b. optic chiasm
   c. lateral geniculate body of the thalamus

14. Fibers from the _____ retinas cross over at the optic chiasm, whereas the _____ fibers do not cross.
   a. temporal; nasal
   b. nasal; temporal
   c. temporal; frontal

15. Lesions in the visual pathway downstream from the optic chiasm damage _____ .
   a. two visual hemifields
   b. only one visual hemifield
   c. none of the visual hemifields

16. When there is a lesion in the _____ , the loss of vision is not a complete hemifield, but a phenomenon called macular sparing takes place, in which the vision in the fovea is spared.
    a. primary visual cortex
    b. visual association area
    c. parietal lobe

17. _____ visual cortical areas deal with the perception of motion of objects and spatial reasoning.
    a. Temporal
    b. Parietal
    c. Occipital

18. _____ visual cortical areas are involved with the complex perception of patterns and forms as recognizable objects.
    a. Parietal
    b. Temporal
    c. Occipital

19. The pretectal area in the _____ mediates the pupillary light reflex, which makes both pupils contract when light enters the retina.
    a. cortex
    b. midbrain
    c. pons

20. If the optic nerve is damaged, _____ or blindness results.
    a. homonymous hemianopsias
    b. anopsia
    c. macular herniation

21. Half-blindness is called _____ .
    a. anopsia
    b. hemianopsia
    c. temporal anopsia

22. Absence of papillary light reflex suggests damage in the _____ .
    a. cortex
    b. brainstem
    c. thalamus

23. If a unilateral dilated pupil does not respond to light, a _____ herniation is suggested.
    a. brainstem
    b. cerebral
    c. cerebellar

24. The primary visual cortex is Brodmann's area _____ .
    a. 19
    b. 18
    c. 17

25. The _____ consists of Brodmann's areas 18 and 19.
    a. primary visual cortex
    b. parietal lobe
    c. visual association cortex

26. The _____ tract is made by projection fibers from the cortex to the oculomotor neurons in the brainstem, which is involved in generating rapid eye movements to objects in the visual field.
    a. corticobasal
    b. corticomesencephalic
    c. corticogeniculate

27. The _____ body is considered the major gateway for visual information into the cortex.
    a. lateral geniculate
    b. medial geniculate
    c. superior geniculate

28. In area 17 the optic radiation synapse contains distinctive white and gray lines and hence it is called the _____ .
    a. corpus striatum
    b. striate cortex
    c. secondary visual area

29. The medial longitudinal fasciculus (MLF) tract carries efferent signals to the _____ nuclei for the control of eye movements.
    a. oculomotor
    b. basal ganglia
    c. vestibular
    d. all of the above
    e. none of the above

II. Matching

1. Superficial sensation
2. Deep sensation
3. Visceral sensations
4. Special senses
5. Adaptation

a. Decrease in rate of discharge of receptors caused by continuous stimulation with constant intensity

b. Touch, pain, temperature, and two-point discrimination

c. Proprioception, deep muscle pain, and vibration sense

d. Hunger, nausea, and pain in the glands

e. Smell, vision, hearing, taste, and equilibrium

III. Fill in the Blanks

Write down at least two signs/symptoms resulting from damage in the following structures.

1. Dorsal column pathways: _____ _____

2. Ventrolateral pathways: _____ _____

3. Damage in the lateral geniculate body: _____ _____

4. Damage at the optic chiasm: _____ _____

5. Damage in the superior colliculus: _____ _____

Answers to Review Questions

I. Multiple Choice

1. b	5. b	9. a	13. b	17. b	21. b	24. c	27. a
2. b	6. b	10. d	14. b	18. c	22. b	25. c	28. b
3. a	7. b	11. c	15. a	19. b	23. a	26. b	29. a
4. c	8. d	12. c	16. c	20. b			

II. Matching

1. b   2. c   3. d   4. e   5. a

III. Fill in the Blanks

1. Deficits in fine discriminative touch sensation, deficits in sense of position in space
2. Phantom limb, hypothermia
3. Homonymous hemianopsia, problems in visual somatosensory system
4. Bitemporal hemianopsia, nasal hemianopsia
5. Inadequate pupillary reflex, abnormal eye movements

Motor Pathways in the Nervous System

After completing this chapter, the learner will:

- **Understand motor pathways and the two major motor tracts called the pyramidal and extrapyramidal tracts.**
- **Explain what constitutes lower and upper motor neurons.**
- **Identify various anatomical levels where motor activities are controlled in the spinal cord, cerebellum, brainstem, basal ganglia, and primary and association motor cortex.**
- **Understand that higher motor centers regulate skilled and patterned movements and involuntary motor activities are controlled by reflex mechanisms.**

Motor Pathways

Clinical Notes

Review Questions

Multiple Choice

MOTOR PATHWAYS

The motor system is an important and very complex component of the nervous system (Figure 9-1). It is responsible for controlling all volitional movements. Damage at any level of the motor system can result in a movement disorder. The descending motor tracts are the neural pathways carrying motor impulses that travel from the cortex to the brainstem and spinal cord. These motor tracts are divided into two categories, depending on their functions. The pyramidal system is a direct motor pathway responsible for controlling voluntary and fine movements. It is called the direct pathway because of its relatively straight course from the cortex to the cranial and spinal nerves (Figure 9-2). The extrapyramidal system is an indirect pathway that controls posture (Figure 9-3). It is called an indirect pathway because of the complex nature of its connections (e.g., the rubrospinal tract). These tracts originate in the basal ganglia and not in the cortex like pyramidal tracts. The pyramidal system works at a conscious level, whereas the extrapyramidal system is more automatic.

Major descending or motor pathways are described in Table 9-1, and differences between pyramidal and extrapyramidal syndromes are shown in Table 9-2.

Functions and locations of motor fibers within specific areas of the nervous system have led to classification of motor neurons. The term *lower motor neuron* (LMN) refers to a motor neuron and its axon in the brainstem or spinal cord. The axon of the LMN innervates a skeletal muscle. Disorders produced by LMN cell body lesions in the spinal cord include amyotrophic lateral sclerosis and poliomyelitis. Lesions in the axon of the LMN lead to denervation of the innervated skeletal muscle fibers and loss of muscle power and precise control. Characteristics of LMN lesions include the following:

1. Wasting
2. Fasciculation
3. Decreased tone (flaccidity)
4. Weakness

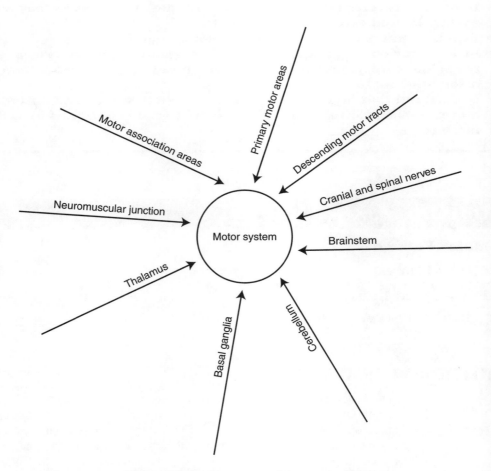

Figure 9-1   Components of the motor system.

5. Decreased or absent reflexes

6. Flexor or absent planter reflexes

The term *upper motor neuron* (UMN) refers to the cell bodies in the motor cortex and their descending axonal processes that synapse on cranial and spinal motor neurons. Characteristics of UMN lesions include the following:

1. No wasting

2. Increased clasp-knife phenomenon

3. Weakness in the antigravity muscles

4. Increased reflexes and clonus

5. Extensor plantar response

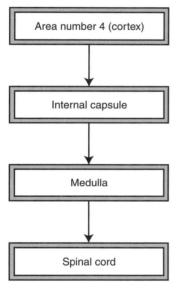

Figure 9-2   Pyramidal tract.

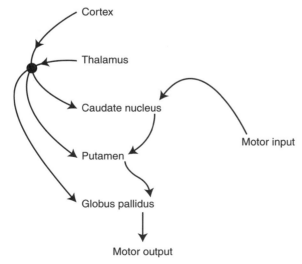

Figure 9-3   Extrapyramidal system showing regulation of motor behaviors.

TABLE 9-1	Course of Motor Pathways

Motor pathways	Origin	Ending
Lateral corticospinal tract	Motor and premotor cortex	Lateral column of spinal cord
Anterior corticospinal tract	Motor and premotor cortex	Anterior column of spinal cord
Vestibulospinal tract	Lateral and medial vestibular nuclei	Ventral column of spinal cord
Rubrospinal tract	Red nucleus of midbrain	Lateral column of spinal cord
Reticulospinal tract	Brainstem	Anterior column of spinal cord
Tectospinal tract	Midbrain	Ventral column of spinal cord

TABLE 9-2	Clinical Signs in Pyramidal and Extrapyramidal Syndromes

Pyramidal syndromes	Extrapyramidal syndromes
Spasticity	Rigidity
Presence of involuntary movements	Absent
Presence of Babinski's sign	Absent
Increased muscle stretch reflexes	Decreased

CLINICAL NOTES

- Amyotrophic lateral sclerosis, also known as Lou Gehrig's disease, is a progressive degenerative condition of the spinal cord and cortical motor neurons characterized by muscular weakness and atrophy.
- Characteristics of primary muscle disease include wasting, weakness, hypotonia, hyporeflexia, and lack of fasciculations.
- Myasthenia gravis is an autoimmune neuromuscular disorder characterized by weakness and fatigability of muscles secondary to the growth of antibodies to acetylcholine receptors.
- Bell's palsy is a common cause of unilateral LMN facial paralysis. Facial weakness develops and there may be pain around the ear or an alteration in facial sensation.
- Bulbar palsy is characterized by bilateral paralysis of the tongue and palate muscles resulting from an LMN disorder. If the paralysis is caused by a bilateral UMN disorder, it is called pseudobulbar palsy (Figure 9-4).

UMN (Figure 9-5) disorders caused by lesions in the cerebral cortex and internal capsule include the following:
- Contralateral hemiplegia, paraplegia, or monoplegia
- Hemianopsia
- Reduced sensations
- Aphasia, agnosia, apraxia, agraphia, and alexia

UMN disorders caused by brainstem lesions include the following:
- Hemiplegia or quadriplegia
- Cranial nerve defects (problems with mastication, facial nerve palsy, vertigo, deafness, nystagmus, dysphagia, and dysarthria)
- Ipsilateral facial sensory impairment
- Loss of pain, temperature, position, vibration changes, and hemianesthesia

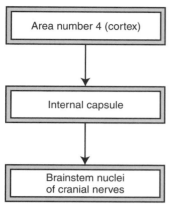

Figure 9-4   Corticobulbar tract.

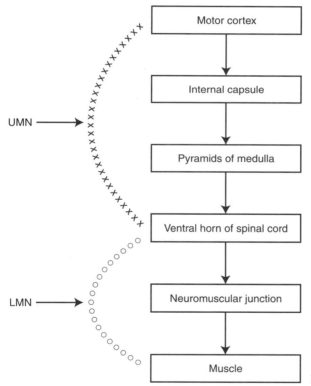

Figure 9-5   UMN and LMN.

UMN disorders caused by lesions in the spinal cord include the following:
- Absence of reflexes/hyporeflexia
- Sensory dissociation
- Ipsilateral paralysis or weakness

- Motor speech disorders (e.g., dysarthria) are speech impairments caused by dysfunction of the motor control centers of the peripheral or central nervous systems or a combination of both. Dysarthria refers to a group of speech disorders characterized by disturbances in a system or in a combination of systems (respiratory, resonatory, phonatory, and articulatory) required for speech. Common speech problems in all kinds of dysarthria include the following:

1. Resonatory problems
2. Phonatory incompetence
3. Articulatory incompetency
4. Prosodic disturbances (excess/insufficiency)
5. Respiratory-phonatory incoordination

The various types of dysarthria are flaccid, spastic, ataxic, hypokinetic, hyperkinetic, and mixed (Figures 9-6 through 9-11).

• Flaccid dysarthria is caused by damage in the cranial nerves, spinal nerves, or neuromuscular junction. It is characterized by muscle weakness that leads to reduced speech intelligibility as a result of various levels of impact on the systems of speech.

• Spastic dysarthria is caused by bilateral damage to the UMN and LMN systems, resulting in spasticity of the muscles required for speech production.

• Ataxic dysarthria is caused by damage to the cerebellum or the cerebellocortical pathways. It is characterized by incoordination of movements of speech muscles.

• Hypokinetic dysarthria is characterized by lesions in the basal ganglia that result in reduced movement of the speech muscles.

• Hyperkinetic dysarthria is also associated with damage in the basal ganglia or extrapyramidal pathways. Involuntary movements interfere mostly with normal speech production.

• Mixed dysarthria occurs when damage is seen in more than one part of the motor system. Mixed dysarthria may be of flaccid-spastic type, hypokinetic-spastic type, etc.

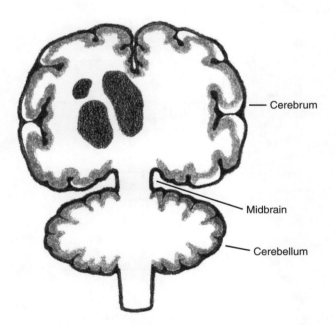

Figure 9-6   Hyperkinetic dysarthria (lesions in putamen, caudate nucleus, and thalamus).

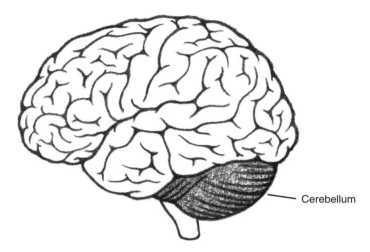

Figure 9-7   Ataxic dysarthria (cerebellar lesions).

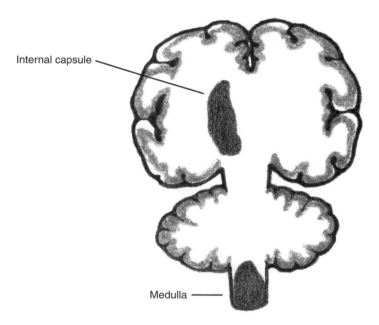

Figure 9-8   Spastic-flaccid dysarthria (lesions in the brainstem and internal capsule).

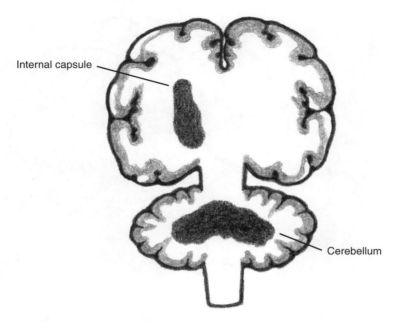

Figure 9-9   Spastic-ataxic dysarthria (lesions in the internal capsule and cerebellum).

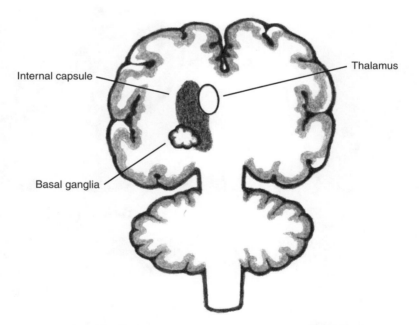

Figure 9-10   Spasticity (lesion in the internal capsule).

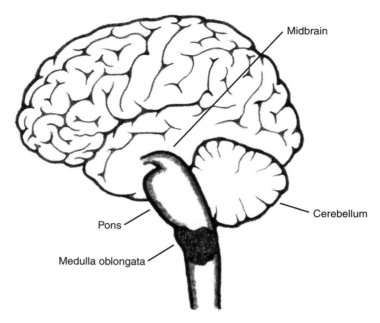

Figure 9-11 Flaccid dysarthria (lesions in the nuclei of cranial nerves IX, X, XI, and XII).

Review Questions

I. Multiple Choice

1. Generalized LMN weakness may result from pathological conditions affecting the lower motor neurons throughout the _____ .
   a. brainstem only
   b. spinal cord and brainstem
   c. spinal cord only

2. Because of involvement of the ocular muscles in myasthenia gravis, _____ , and _____ are seen.
   a. ptosis; diplopia
   b. nystagmus; decreased papillary reflex
   c. neither of the above

3. Involvement of bulbar muscles causes _____ and _____ .
   a. dysarthria; dysphagia
   b. dysphasia; trunk weakness
   c. dysnomia; limb weakness

4. The pyramidal pathway is also called the _____ pathway.
   a. direct
   b. indirect
   c. neither of the above

5. The extrapyramidal pathway is also called the _____ pathway.
   a. direct
   b. indirect
   c. neither of the above

6. The _____ tract is part of the pyramidal system.
   a. corticobasal
   b. corticospinal
   c. corticothalamic
   d. corticopontine
   e. corticomedullary

7. Lesions of the internal capsule are more likely to produce complete hemiparesis, whereas _____ lesions are more likely to affect just the hand, leg, or face.
   a. cortical
   b. subcortical
   c. brainstem
   d. none of the above

8. _____ is a sign of LMN damage.
   a. Hyperreflexia
   b. Atrophy
   c. Spasticity
   d. Rigidity

9. Damage in the corticospinal tract might result in _____ .
   a. sensory loss
   b. muscular dystrophy
   c. paralysis of the limbs
   d. none of the above

10. Increased tension in the muscle caused by imbalance between alpha and gamma motor neurons is found in _____ .
    a. spasticity
    b. flaccidity
    c. rigidity
    d. a and b
    e. none of the above

11. Increased tone caused by extrapyramidal tract pathological conditions that is characterized by steady resistance to passive motion is found in _____ .
    a. spasticity
    b. rigidity
    c. a and b
    d. none of the above

12. _____ neurons are motor neurons in the cranial and spinal nerves.
    a. LMN
    b. UMN
    c. Both UMN and LMN
    d. None of the above

13. Damage to the UMN results in _____ .
    a. spasticity
    b. flaccidity
    c. rigidity
    d. atrophy

14. The _____ is the point where the axons of the LMN make specific connections with muscle cells.
    a. brainstem
    b. neuromuscular junction
    c. synapse
    d. none of the above

15. During LMN paralysis the gradual loss of tissue in the affected muscle is called

    _____ .
    a. muscular paresis
    b. muscular paralysis
    c. muscular dystrophy

16. _____ is an infectious viral disease that attacks the cell bodies of the
    LMN.
    a. Tumor
    b. Polio
    c. Amyotrophic lateral sclerosis

17. _____ is a disorder that can affect both the UMN and the LMN. When
    LMNs are affected, it results in _____ dysarthria.
    a. Progressive supranuclear palsy; spastic
    b. Progressive bulbar palsy; flaccid
    c. Progressive bulbar palsy; spastic

18. The speech characteristics of flaccid dysarthria include _____ .
    a. hypernasality
    b. nasal emission
    c. imprecise articulation
    d. phonatory-respiratory incompetence
    e. all of the above

19. Motor deficits in spastic dysarthria are caused by bilateral damage to the _____
    _____ tracts.
    a. UMN
    b. LMN
    c. a and b
    d. none of the above

20. Damage to the parts of the _____ system serving the speech mechanism
    will result in weakness and slowness in speech musculature.
    a. extrapyramidal
    b. pyramidal
    c. cerebellar

21. _____ is an immunologic disorder that results in destruction of the
    myelin sheath in the cerebral hemispheres, cerebellum, brainstem, and spinal cord. This
    disorder may result in spastic, ataxic, and mixed dysarthria.
    a. Myasthenia gravis
    b. Multiple sclerosis
    c. Huntington's chorea

22. A large bundle of myelinated axons called the _____ tract descends from Brodmann's areas 4 and 6 through the brainstem and then decussates downward into the lateral white columns of the spinal cord.
    a. corticobasal
    b. corticopontine
    c. corticospinal
    d. corticothalamic

23. The _____ of the spinal cord control muscular contractions via lower motor neurons.
    a. posterior horn cells
    b. anterior horn cells
    c. neither of the above

24. The area in the brainstem where the great majority of axons in the corticospinal system decussate is called the _____ .
    a. pontine pyramid
    b. medullary pyramid
    c. cortical pyramid
    d. none of the above

Answers to Review Questions

I. Multiple Choice

1. b	4. a	7. a	10. a	13. a	16. b	19. a	22. c
2. a	5. b	8. b	11. c	14. b	17. a	20. a	23. b
3. a	6. b	9. c	12. c	15. c	18. e	21. b	24. b

10

Disorders of the Cerebral Cortex

OBJECTIVES

After completing this chapter, the learner will:

- Know which cortical and subcortical centers are needed to process speech and language.
- Be able to describe the clinical features of aphasia, apraxia, agnosia, and amnesia, which are disorders of the cerebral cortex.

OUTLINE

CORTICAL AND SUBCORTICAL CENTERS

The major cortical centers for speech and language seen on the brain's lateral surface include Broca's area, Wernicke's area, postcentral gyrus, precentral gyrus, supramarginal gyrus, and angular gyrus. The major centers for speech and language seen on the medial surface of the brain include the cingular gyrus and corpus callosum. The major subcortical centers for speech and language seen in the coronal section of the brain include the basal ganglia nuclei (caudate nucleus, putamen, and globus pallidus), substantia nigra, and red nucleus. Specific speech areas on the brain correspond to Broca's area (Brodmann's areas 44 and 45), motor cortex, extrapyramidal and pyramidal tracts, subcortical nuclei (basal ganglia, brainstem, cerebellum, and related cranial and spinal nerves). Refer to Table 3-1 for an outline of the main lobes of the brain and their functions.

Some of the major types of neurological disorders that affect the cerebral cortex include neurogenetic diseases (e.g., Huntington's disease), developmental disorders (e.g., cerebral palsy), degenerative diseases of adult life (e.g., Alzheimer's and Parkinson's disease), metabolic diseases (Wilson's disease), cerebrovascular diseases (e.g., stroke, vascular dementia), convulsive disorders (e.g., epilepsy), and infectious diseases (e.g., acquired immune deficiency syndrome). All these disorders are covered in the review questions section.

CLINICAL NOTES

Cortical/Subcortical Disorders

Aphasias

- Broca aphasia: Broca's area (Figure 10-1); nonfluent, dysprosody, agrammatic and telegraphic speech, good comprehension, poor repetition, and naming depends on impairment
- Wernicke's aphasia (Figure 10-2): Wernicke's area; good fluency, poor comprehension and repetition, naming depends on impairment, jargon
- Global aphasia (Figure 10-3): Entire perisylvian zone (anterior and posterior); nonfluent, poor comprehension, poor naming and repetition

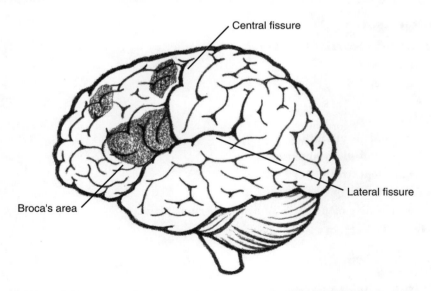

Figure 10-1   Expressive aphasia with mild dyspraxia (lesions in Broca's area and motor areas).

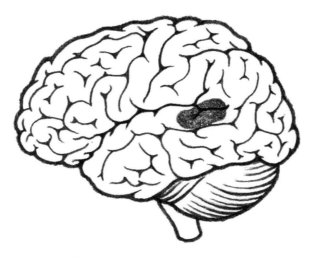

Figure 10-2 Wernicke's aphasia.

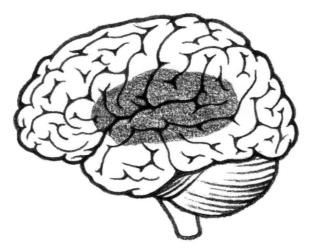

Figure 10-3 Global aphasia (lesion in the perisylvian zone).

- Transcortical motor aphasia (Figure 10-4): Areas anterior to Broca's area; nonfluent, good comprehension and repetition, naming depends on impairment
- Transcortical sensory aphasia (Figure 10-5): Areas posterior to Wernicke's area; good fluency and repetition, poor comprehension, naming depends on impairment
- Conduction aphasia (Figure 10-6): Arcuate fasciculus; good fluency and comprehension, poor repetition, naming depends on impairment
- Anomia: Posterior/anterior cerebral lesions; good fluency, comprehension, and repetition; poor naming

Apraxias (parietal lobe lesions)

- Ideational: Disruption of ideas to understand the use of objects
- Ideomotor: Disruption of plans needed to demonstrate actions
- Speech: Slow effortful speech, inconsistent errors, often seen with Broca's

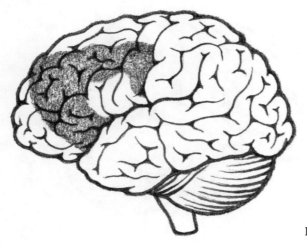

Figure 10-4   Transcortical motor aphasias.

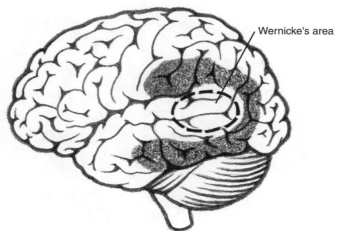

Wernicke's area

Figure 10-5   Transcortical sensory aphasia.

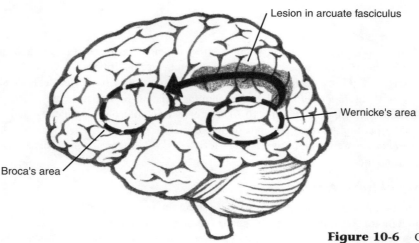

Lesion in arcuate fasciculus

Wernicke's area

Broca's area

Figure 10-6   Conduction aphasia.

Agnosias

- Visual agnosia (Figure 10-7): Occipital lobe damage; problems in shape recognition, inability to copy drawings, inability to recognize faces (prosopagnosia), inability to recognize what is being copied, difficulty in transforming visual information to verbal mechanisms
- Auditory agnosia (Figure 10-8): Temporal lobe damage; inability to interpret auditory stimuli despite normal peripheral hearing
- Tactile agnosia (Figure 10-9): Parietal lobe damage; inability to name objects using tactile modality

Dysarthrias

- Ataxic: Cerebellar damage; monotonous pitch, speech timing and articulatory problems, harsh vocal quality
- Flaccid: Lower motor neuron (LMN) damage; hypernasality, breathy voice, imprecise consonant production

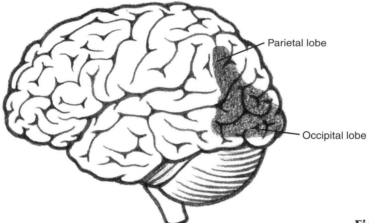

Figure 10-7   Visual agnosia.

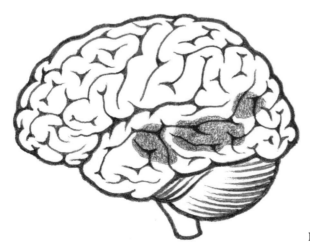

Figure 10-8   Auditory agnosia.

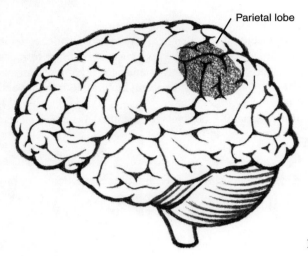

Parietal lobe

Figure 10-9   Tactile agnosia.

- Hyperkinetic: Extrapyramidal system damage; excessive involuntary movements, abnormal muscle tone
- Hypokinetic: Extrapyramidal system damage; slow movements, monotonous pitch and loudness, reduced stress, imprecise consonants
- Spastic: Bilateral upper motor neuron (UMN) damage; imprecise articulation, monotonous pitch and loudness, poor prosody, sluggish, stiff muscles

Traumatic brain injury

Cortical and/or subcortical lesions, lacerations, contusions, and concussions; problems in planning, problem solving, attention, memory, visual processing, deeper language, and pragmatics

Right hemisphere syndrome

Right hemisphere damage; agnosia, left hemispatial neglect, visuoperceptual and attentional impairments

Brainstem stroke

Brainstem lesions; flaccid dysarthria, weak voice, intact language, dysphagia

Pseudobulbar palsy

Medullary damage; spastic dysarthria, spatial/perceptual impairment, confusion and disorientation

Degenerative or progressive neuromuscular diseases

- Myasthenia gravis: Neuromuscular junction lesion; fatigable weakness of skeletal muscles, failure of neuromuscular transmission, dysphagia
- Amyotrophic lateral sclerosis: Degeneration of the UMNs and LMNs; dysphagia and dysarthria
- Parkinson's disease: Degeneration of the basal ganglia or substantia nigra; bradykinesia (slow movement), rigidity, tremor, and loss of postural reflexes, dysphagia
- Huntington's chorea: Extrapyramidal tracts damage; progresses into dementia, no inhibition of movements, dysphagia
- Alzheimer's disease: Cortical lesions; memory loss, anomia, intellectual deterioration, motor speech progressing to rigidity, dysphagia
- Progressive supranuclear palsy: Pyramidal and extrapyramidal tract lesion; hyperkinetic or spastic-ataxic dysarthria, intellectual deterioration, dysphagia

Review Questions

I. Matching

Match the following disorders with the sites of their lesions.
 1. Flaccid dysarthria
 2. Spastic dysarthria
 3. Hyperkinetic dysarthria
 4. Wernicke's aphasia
 5. Ataxic dysarthria
 6. Subcortical aphasia
 7. Parkinson's disease
 8. Broca's aphasia
 9. Amyotrophic lateral sclerosis
10. Pseudobulbar palsy

a. Medulla
b. UMN and LMN
c. Anterior perisylvian area
d. Thalamus
e. Substantia nigra
f. Cerebellum
g. UMN
h. Area 22
i. LMN
j. Extrapyramidal system

II. Matching

Match the following disease descriptions with the conditions listed.
 1. Damage to the brain caused by arterial blockage that produces a condition that is one of the most common causes of death in United States.
 2. One of the most common causes of stroke.
 3. A local ballooning out of an arterial wall.
 4. Berry aneurysms are located around this structure.
 5. A congenital anomaly with tangled veins and arteries with no capillaries.
 6. A spasm or occlusion of an artery causing temporary neurological deficits lasting minutes or hours followed by complete recovery of function.
 7. Usually the arachnoid membrane and the pia mater are affected in this type of bacterial infection.

8. Pockets of pus in the brain tissue formed as the result of bacterial infection.
9. The tertiary condition of this disease causes mental disorders.
10. Caused by viral infections leading to LMN paralysis.
11. An infection in the brain tissue caused by viral attacks.
12. Characterized by behavioral and cognitive changes such as apathy and memory loss.
13. A disease transmitted via an animal bite that causes hydrophobia, laryngeal spasms, excitability, and convulsions.
14. Intermittent weakness and fatigability of voluntary muscles resulting from an autoimmune disease and causing dysphonia and dysphagia.
15. Injury to the CNS caused by accidents and violence resulting in closed or open head injury.

a. Brain abscess
b. Syphilis
c. Embolus
d. Rabies
e. Circle of Willis
f. Stroke
g. Aneurysm
h. Arteriovenous malformation
i. Transient ischemic attack
j. Encephalitis
k. Meningitis
l. Myasthenia gravis
m. Traumatic brain injury
n. Dementia
o. Poliomyelitis

III. Multiple Choice

1. _____ is a type of subcortical dementia.
   a. Huntington's disease
   b. Pick's disease
   c. Alzheimer's disease

2. _____ is one of the CT/MRI findings in dementia.
   a. Tumor
   b. Meningeal abscess
   c. Dilation of ventricles

3. Injury caused by _____ acceleration is more severe than _____

   _____ acceleration.
   a. angular; linear
   b. linear; angular
   c. neither of the above

4. _____ is used to assess coma in acute traumatic brain injury patients.
   a. Glasgow coma scale
   b. Colored progressive matrices test
   c. Mini mental state examination

5. Jargon is commonly seen in _____ aphasia.
   a. posterior
   b. anterior
   c. subcortical

6. Visual imperception and agnosias are caused by impairment in the _____ .
   a. temporal lobe
   b. occipital lobe
   c. frontal lobe

7. In Alzheimer's disease, blood vessels are _____ .
   a. constricted
   b. dilated
   c. a and b
   d. none of the above

8. _____ is a buildup of fatty deposits, particularly cholesterol.
   a. CVA
   b. Aneurysm
   c. Arteriosclerosis

9. The most common type of stroke is caused by _____ .
   a. blockage
   b. bleeding
   c. headache
   d. none of the above

10. New blood vessels can grow in the area of the brain after a _____ stroke.
    a. minor
    b. major
    c. neither of the above

11. Obstruction of one or more arteries that supply blood to the brain results in _____

    _____ .
    a. cerebrovascular insufficiency
    b. arteriovenous malformations
    c. aneurysms

12. _____ is the blockage of a vessel caused by dislodged clot, tumor cells, etc.
    a. Embolism
    b. Thrombosis
    c. Aneurysm

13. The most common locations for _____ are in the region of the anterior communicating and anterior cerebral arteries.
    a. embolism
    b. aneurysm
    c. clots

14. A _____ lesion leads to loss of muscle contraction for reflexes and voluntary activities, hypotonia, muscle atrophy, and fasciculation.
    a. brainstem
    b. myoneural junction
    c. muscle fiber
    d. none of the above

15. A lesion in the _____ leads to weakness and increased fatigability over a short time period.
    a. brainstem
    b. myoneural junction
    c. muscle fibers

16. A lesion in the _____ leads to hypertrophy of muscles, failure to contract, and formation of fibrosis.
    a. brainstem
    b. myoneural junction
    c. muscle fibers

17. A history of high blood pressure is likely to cause sudden losses of consciousness, which leads to loss of the ability to move or speak. The diagnosis is likely to be _____ .
    a. a meningioma
    b. Alzheimer's disease
    c. Wallerian degeneration
    d. a and b
    e. none of the above

18. Alzheimer's disease is characterized by _____ .
    a. gliosis
    b. depigmentation of the substantia nigra
    c. neurofibrillary tangles and senile neuritic plaques
    d. all of the above
    e. none of the above

19. The most significant outcome of the Arnold-Chiari malformation is _____ .
    a. muscle paralysis
    b. aneurysm
    c. hemorrhage

20. A patient involved in a motor vehicle accident complained of headaches, irritability, and other personality problems. The diagnosis is likely to be _____ .
    a. cerebellar damage
    b. cerebral concussion
    c. acoustic neuroma

21. An MRI scan of a patient with a prolonged history of alcoholism indicated atrophy of the cerebellum. The patient is likely to show _____ .
    a. apraxia
    b. ataxia
    c. agnosia

22. An insufficient supply of oxygen leads to a condition called _____ .
    a. necrosis
    b. hypoxia
    c. ganglionitis

23. _____ atrophy is the most common atrophy seen in Alzheimer's disease.
    a. Diffuse
    b. Focal
    c. Frontal

24. In classical _____ there is a characteristic asymmetrical frontotemporal lobe permanent brain atrophy pattern.
    a. Pick's disease
    b. Alzheimer's disease
    c. normal aging

25. In _____ a clinical triad of ataxia, ophthalmoplegia, and mental confusion are seen.
    a. methanol poisoning
    b. central pontine myelinosis
    c. Wernicke's encephalopathy

26. Right hemisphere impairments may result in _____ .
    a. anosognosia
    b. difficulty in organization
    c. left neglect
    d. all the above
    e. none of the above

27. The causes of cerebrovascular accident are _____ .
    a. thrombosis
    b. hypertension
    c. embolism
    d. all of the above

28. _____ is the inability to recognize stimuli through an intact sensory modality.
    a. Aphasia
    b. Agnosia
    c. Apraxia

29. The pathophysiology of multiple sclerosis includes _____ .
    a. formation of glial scar tissues
    b. degeneration of white matter tracts
    c. degeneration of myelin sheath
    d. all of the above

30. The principal pathological aspects in _____ are decreased excitation and contraction of muscles.
    a. myasthenia gravis
    b. multiple sclerosis
    c. Pick's disease
    d. none of the above

31. Possible etiology in myasthenia gravis is _____ .
    a. abnormal distribution of the receptors at the neuromuscular junction
    b. insufficient production of receptor proteins
    c. abnormality in the neurotransmitters
    d. none of the above
    e. all of the above

32. Traditionally brain injuries have been classified as mild, moderate, and severe based on length of the time of loss of _____ .
    a. language functions
    b. speech
    c. consciousness

33. _____ adequately predicts the amount of tissue damage caused by traumatic brain injury.
    a. Loss of language
    b. Duration of coma
    c. Loss of cognition
    d. None of the above

34. Because of rapid deceleration of vehicles in a crash, the brain is subjected to shearing forces that tear or stretch the _____ .
    a. dendrites
    b. axon
    c. cell bodies

35. Copper being transported in the blood may be deposited in the liver, basal ganglia, and cerebellum in _____ disease.
    a. Wilson's
    b. Pick's
    c. Alzheimer's
    d. None of the above

36. The dysarthrias seen in Wilson's disease are _____ .
    a. ataxic-spastic
    b. hyperkinetic
    c. hypokinetic
    d. a and b
    e. all of the above

37. The pathophysiology of Parkinson's disease includes _____ .
    a. depigmentation and degeneration of substantia niagra
    b. degeneration of globus pallidus
    c. reduction of dopamine
    d. all of the above

38. _____ is very common in Parkinson's disease.
    a. Bradykinesia
    b. Tremors during sleep
    c. Tremor of the head and face

39. The histological hallmarks of Alzheimer's disease include _____ .
    a. neurofibrillary tangles
    b. amyloid plaques
    c. a and b
    d. none of the above

40. A patient was diagnosed with left-sided paralysis and neglect syndrome. The possible diagnosis is _____ .
    a. right hemisphere damage
    b. left hemisphere damage
    c. both a and b
    d. none of the above

41. _____ refers to loss of memory.
    a. Amnesia
    b. Agnosia
    c. Anomia
    d. Apraxia

42. Memory loss usually results from _____ damage to parts of the brain vital for memory storage, processing, or recall.
    a. unilateral
    b. bilateral
    c. partial

43. _____ is a neurological disorder caused by disturbances in normal electrical functions in the brain.
    a. Huntington's chorea
    b. Epilepsy
    c. Myoclonus

44. There are two main types of epileptic seizures: _____ and generalized.
    a. partial
    b. complex
    c. simple

45. Homonymous hemianopsias most commonly result from pathological conditions of the white matter in the _____ .
    a. parietal and upper temporal lobes
    b. occipital lobe
    c. frontal lobe

46. _____ is a rare disorder characterized by an inability to recognize and identify objects or persons despite having knowledge of the same.
    a. Apraxia
    b. Agnosia
    c. Aphasia
    d. None of the above

Answers to Review Questions

Matching

1. i	3. j	5. f	7. e	9. b
2. g	4. h	6. d	8. c	10. a

Matching

1. f	3. g	5. h	7. k	9. b	11. j	13. d	15. m
2. c	4. e	6. i	8. a	10. o	12. n	14. l

III. Multiple Choice

1. a	7. a	13. b	19. c	25. c	31. e	37. d	43. b
2. c	8. c	14. b	20. b	26. d	32. c	38. a	44. a
3. a	9. a	15. b	21. b	27. d	33. b	39. c	45. a
4. a	10. a	16. c	22. b	28. b	34. b	40. a	46. b
5. a	11. a	17. e	23. a	29. d	35. a	41. a	
6. b	12. a	18. d	24. a	30. a	36. d	42. b	

11

Neurological Assessments

OUTLINE OF CASE HISTORY FOR NEUROLOGICAL EXAMINATION

1. Information from the patient and family and referral information
2. Present complaint, onset, progression, and symptoms of illness
3. Past history of any medical problems and medications

NEUROLOGICAL EXAMINATION

1. Level of consciousness
2. Cognitive status (attention; alertness; orientation to time, person, and place; short-term and long-term memory; problem-solving and abstract reasoning ability)
3. Mood, affect, and behaviors
4. Language (receptive and expressive levels; content, form, and use)
5. Speech patterns (spontaneous speech, fluency, speech intelligibility, etc.)
6. Integrity of sensory processes (visual, tactile, auditory, and kinesthetic systems)
7. Integrity of motor processes (neuromuscular control over speech systems—respiration, phonation, articulation, and prosody)
8. Cranial nerve examination

Review Questions

I. Matching

Match the following neurodiagnostic tools with their appropriate descriptions.

1. MRI
2. Angiography
3. EMG
4. PET
5. EEG

a. Recording of electrical impulses in the muscles
b. Recording of electrical impulses in the brain
c. Recording of cerebral metabolism
d. Radiographic visualization of blood vessels
e. Magnetic nuclei in a patient are aligned in a strong magnetic field to capture three-dimensional (3-D) images

II. Matching

Match the following disease conditions with the appropriate neurodiagnostic method.

1. Hydrocephalus
2. Lower motor neuron disease
3. Midline brain structures
4. Aneurysms
5. Blood flow
6. Tumor in the spinal cord
7. Seizures
8. Infarctions

a. Myelography
b. Electroencephalography
c. Electromyography
d. Ultrasonography
e. Angiography
f. Magnetic resonance imaging
g. Positron-emission tomography
h. Computed tomography

III. Matching

Match the following neurodiagnostic findings with the appropriate disease conditions.

1. Denervation patterns with fibrillation potentials
2. Degeneration of substantia nigra
3. Reduced action potential from skeletal muscles
4. Sclerotic plaques
5. Cerebral atrophy
6. Dural laceration
7. Compression and destruction of nervous tissue
8. Abdominal electrical discharge in a focal point

a. Parkinson's disease
b. Myasthenia gravis
c. Alzheimer's disease
d. Traumatic brain injury
e. Brain tumor
f. Seizure
g. Alzheimer's disease
h. Multiple sclerosis

IV. Multiple Choice

1. In the _____ examination, level of consciousness is tested.
   a. mentation
   b. cognitive status
   c. motor

2. The cognitive status examination includes all of the following except _____ .
   a. memory
   b. orientation
   c. problem solving
   d. social adjustments

3. Spontaneous speech, word usage, fluency, and information content are components of _____ examination.
   a. motor
   b. cognition
   c. language

4. _____ testing includes testing of insights, judgments, abstract, and concrete thinking.
   a. Speech
   b. Mental status
   c. Language

5. _____ testing is an important component of the neurological examination.
   a. Intelligence quotient
   b. Personality
   c. Cranial nerve

6. Integrity of the _____ lobe is tested to measure superficial and deep sensations.
   a. temporal
   b. parietal
   c. frontal

7. In the cognitive status examination, it is important to _____ .
   a. estimate premorbid intellectual levels
   b. test immediate memory
   c. test integrity of thought process
   d. all of the above

8. Patients diagnosed with aphasia, disorientation, and amnesia show problems with _____
   a. fund of knowledge
   b. level of consciousness
   c. memory

9. Some of the speech and language disturbances found in left-hemisphere syndrome include

   all of the following except _____ .
   a. prosopagnosia
   b. impaired comprehension
   c. paraphasias
   d. effortful speech

10. Speech and language disorders commonly occur in neurological diseases and hence exami-

    nation is needed to determine the presence of _____ .
    a. dysarthria
    b. apraxia
    c. aphasia
    d. all of the above

11. An absence of plantar reflex indicates a _____ lesion.
    a. brainstem
    b. corticospinal tract
    c. spinal segmental lesion

12. Ptosis is observed secondary to paresis or paralysis of cranial nerves _____ .
    a. III and IV
    b. III and VI
    c. III, IV, and VI

13. Absence of _____ reflex is found in oculomotor nerve or midbrain lesions.
    a. startle
    b. pupillary
    c. accommodation

14. A lesion in the _____ lobe results in loss of voluntary conjugate eye
    movements.
    a. parietal
    b. frontal
    c. temporal

15. Loss of tracking movements of the eyes is caused by a lesion in the _____
    lobe.
    a. frontal
    b. temporal
    c. occipital

16. Decrease or loss of corneal reflex is caused by a _____ lesion.
    a. peripheral
    b. brainstem
    c. both a and b

17. Paralysis of the lower face indicates a _____ lesion.
    a. contralateral cerebral hemisphere
    b. brainstem
    c. both a and b

18. Vagal nerve disorder include all of the following except _____ .
    a. dysphonia
    b. nasal regurgitation
    c. aspiration
    d. tongue atrophy

19. Weak shoulder shrug and head turning indicate a disorder in cranial nerve _____

    _____ .

    a. IX
    b. X
    c. XI

20. A paroxysmal pain radiating from the throat to the ear indicates a _____
    cranial nerve lesion.
    a. tenth
    b. ninth
    c. twelfth

21. Unilateral or bilateral flaccid paralysis of the tongue indicates a lesion of the _____

    _____ cranial nerve.

    a. seventh
    b. twelfth
    c. ninth

22. Fasciculations of the tongue muscles are seen in _____ dysarthria.
    a. ataxic
    b. flaccid
    c. spastic

23. _____ refers to the loss of muscle bulk secondary to a peripheral lesion.
    a. Atrophy
    b. Spasticity
    c. Flaccidity

24. _____ refers to a compensatory response to weakness caused by damaged
    muscle groups.
    a. Fasciculation
    b. Atrophy
    c. Hypertrophy

25. Decreased muscle tone or _____ indicates cerebellar proprioceptive
    impairment.
    a. atonia
    b. hypertonia
    c. hypotonia

26. Cogwheel-type rigidity is found in _____ .
    a. Parkinson's disease
    b. flaccid cerebral palsy
    c. myasthenia gravis

27. _____ is the inability to perform coordinated movements.
    a. Dysmetria
    b. Ataxia
    c. Atonia

28. Inability to perform rapid alternating movements is called _____ .
    a. dysdiadochokinesia
    b. clasp-knife phenomenon
    c. ballismus

29. Scissored gait is observed in _____ lesions.
    a. bilateral reticular tract
    b. unilateral corticobulbar tract
    c. bilateral corticospinal tract

30. A positive Romberg sign is seen in _____ lesions.
    a. dorsal column
    b. ventral column
    c. neither of the above

31. Purposeless, rhythmic movements of various body parts (head, limbs, face) are called

    _____ .
    a. fasciculations
    b. fibrillations
    c. tremors

32. Resting tremors are caused by lesions in the _____ .
    a. spinal cord
    b. basal ganglia
    c. cerebellum

33. Causalgias or burning pain is the result of _____ nerve irritation.
    a. cranial
    b. peripheral
    c. neither of the above

34. _____ refers to nonrhythmic, rapid, jerky movements caused by corticospinal tract or other central lesions.
    a. Tic
    b. Dyskinesia
    c. Myoclonus

35. Lesions in the parietal lobe lead to all of the following conditions except _____
    _____ .
    a. astereognosis
    b. loss of two-point discrimination
    c. loss of tactile sensations
    d. dyskinesia

36. Upper motor neuron syndromes are characterized by _____ .
    a. increased deep tendon reflexes
    b. decreased superficial reflexes
    c. spasticity
    d. all of the above

37. Lesions above the medulla affect the _____ side of the body.
    a. ipsilateral
    b. contralateral
    c. neither of the above

38. _____ lesions are characterized by hyporeflexia, areflexia, flaccidity, atrophy, and fasciculations.
    a. Sensory neuron
    b. Lower motor neuron
    c. Upper motor neuron

39. Computerized reconstructions of sections of the head and body after passing x-ray beams through them are called _____ .
    a. positron-emission tomograms
    b. computed tomograms
    c. angiograms

40. The neurodiagnostic method in which the patient is placed in a static magnetic field and the computer is used to create images of the structures is called _____ .
    a. positron-emission tomography
    b. computed tomography
    c. magnetic resonance imaging

41. Use of ultrasonic energy to examine midline structures is called _____ .
    a. computed tomography
    b. ultrasonography
    c. angiography

42. In the _____ method, electrical impulses generated by the brain are received by electrodes placed on the surface of the head.
    a. electroencephalographic
    b. electropalatographic
    c. electromyographic

43. _____ uses positron-emitting radionuclear materials to measure cerebral metabolism, blood flow, and other cellular structures.
    a. Positron-emission tomography
    b. Computed tomography
    c. Angiography

44. _____ refers to the recording of electrical changes in muscle fibers.
    a. Electromyography
    b. Electroencephalography
    c. None of the above

45. Radiographic visualization of arteries and veins in the brain is done with _____

    _____ .
    a. electromyography
    b. myelography
    c. angiography

46. _____ is used to visualize the spinal canal and the subarachnoid space by x-ray and fluoroscopy.
    a. Angiography
    b. Myelography
    c. Electromyography

47. Abnormal electrical activities in the brain may be caused by _____ .
    a. seizures
    b. head injury
    c. stroke
    d. aneurysms
    e. all of the above

V. Fill in the Blanks

In the following spaces, indicate the purposes of the following neurodiagnostic procedures.

1. CAT scan _____

2. PET _____

3. MRI _____

4. Ultrasonography _____

5. EEG _____

6. EMG _____

7. Myelography _____

8. Angiography _____

9. Spinal tap _____

VI. True or False

1. Space-occupying lesions in the cerebrum may be detected by angiography.
2. The magnetic resonance imaging method uses x-ray beams.
3. Ultrasonography is a noninvasive procedure.
4. Central metabolism may be measured by MRI.
5. EEG can detect tumors in the brain.
6. Electromyography may be used to diagnose sensory deficits secondary to brain damage.
7. Stenosis of arteries is detected by cerebral angiography.
8. Tumors of the spinal cord are detected easily by EEG.
9. Nerve conduction times slow down with age.
10. Diseases of the neuromuscular junction are diagnosed with EMG.
11. A neurologist uses the patient's complaints and medical history, the neurological examination, and specific neurodiagnostic/laboratory tests to arrive at a diagnosis.
12. Hereditary diseases (e.g., Huntington's disease) do not have a definite genetic inheritance pattern.
13. Understanding the pattern of symptom development is very important for diagnosing a progressive disease condition (e.g., multiple sclerosis).
14. Patients with damage in the motor cortex usually complain of generalized weakness on both sides of the body.
15. Patients with basal ganglia damage usually complain of lack of muscle tone.
16. Muscle atrophy suggests upper motor neuron pathology.
17. Patients with Parkinson's disease usually complain of hyperesthesia or abnormal sensitivity to stimulation.
18. Sensory loss in one side of the body suggests damage in the ascending spinal cord tracts or the sensory cortex.
19. A positive Romberg's sign is noted when patients become unsteady while their eyes are closed.
20. Caloric testing is used to rule out auditory pathology.
21. Patients with acute confusional state usually have no problem with orientation.
22. Amnestic states are a frequent consequence of traumatic brain injury.
23. Syncope denotes transitory loss of consciousness caused by a brief reduction of blood supply to the brain.

Answers to Review Questions

I. Matching

1. e   2. d   3. a   4. c   5. b

II. Matching

1. h   2. e   3. d   4. e   5. g   6. a   7. b   8. f

III. Matching

1. c   2. a   3. b   4. h   5. g   6. d   7. e   8. f

IV. Multiple Choice

1. a	7. d	13. b	19. c	25. c	31. c	37. b	43. a
2. d	8. c	14. b	20. b	26. a	32. b	38. b	44. a
3. c	9. a	15. a	21. b	27. b	33. b	39. b	45. c
4. b	10. d	16. b	22. b	28. a	34. b	40. c	46. b
5. c	11. b	17. b	23. a	29. c	35. d	41. b	47. e
6. b	12. a	18. d	24. a	30. a	36. d	42. a	

V. Fill in the Blanks

1. CAT scan: Also called CT scan; used to visualize sectional anatomy of both external and internal structures in the nervous system; computerized images are formed with the help of intravenous contrast agents.

2. PET: Used to measure glucose and oxygen metabolism along with cerebral blood flow.

3. MRI: Used to study structures that are not quite captured by CT scans; computerized images are formed with the help of magnetic fields.

4. Ultrasonography: Used to locate midline brain structures for the purpose of diagnosing intracranial abnormalities.

5. EEG: Used to localize anatomic pathological conditions in cases of abnormal cerebral function that cannot be visualized radiographically or magnetically (e.g., transient states such as seizures); records electrical impulses generated by the brain that are received by electrodes on the surface of the scalp.

6. EMG: Used to understand pathological conditions related to peripheral nerves and muscular disorders; records spontaneous, voluntary, and electrically stimulated muscle activities and action potentials of muscle fibers.

7. Myelography: Used to visualize the spinal cord and subarachnoid space.

8. Angiography: Used to visualize intracranial and extracranial circulation and blood vessels, in particular, to detect various vascular pathological conditions.

9. Spinal tap: Procedure by which cerebrospinal fluid is extracted from the spinal cord for purposes of analysis to detect various pathological conditions of the nervous system.

VI. True or False

1. False	5. True	9. True	13. True	17. False	21. False
2. False	6. False	10. True	14. False	18. True	22. True
3. True	7. True	11. True	15. False	19. True	23. True
4. False	8. False	12. False	16. False	20. False	

12

Developmental Neurology: Part I

OBJECTIVES

After completing this chapter, the learner will:

- **Recognize that the nervous system is highly organized with a complex network of neural connections.**
- **Understand that the maturation of the nervous system is also a complex process embedded in a series of biological changes.**

OUTLINE

NEUROEMBRYOLOGY

Briefly, the sequence of development of the nervous system is as follows:

1. Thickening of the dorsomedial part of ectoderm leads to the formation of neuroderm (also called the neural plate).

2. The mesoderm forms a rodlike structure called the notochord, which serves as a vertebral skeleton for the embryo.

3. The lateral margins of the neural plate elevate, creating depressions called neural folds or grooves.

4. Neural folds move medially to form a closed tube called the neural tube.

5. Portions of the neural folds that do not participate in forming the neural tube form a structure called the neural crest.

6. The central nervous system, consisting of the brain and spinal cord, is derived from the neural tube.

7. The peripheral nervous system is derived from the neural crest.

8. Three primary vesicles develop from the neural tube: the rhombencephalon, mesencephalon, and prosencephalon

9. The rhombencephalon divides into the myelencephalon (medulla oblongata) and the metencephalon (pons and cerebellum).

10. The mesencephalon does not divide, but the prosencephalon subdivides into the diencephalon (epithalamus, thalamus, and hypothalamus) and the telencephalon at the origin of the basal forebrain and cerebral hemispheres.

11. From the telencephalon, a pair of vesicles develop that eventually become the right and left hemispheres.

12. The ventricles, which contain the cerebrospinal fluid, are also derived from the neural tube.

13. The meninges that form around the neural tube (pia mater, arachnoid membrane, and dura mater) are derived from the mesoderm.

14. From the wall of the neural tube, neuroblasts, which are undifferentiated nerve cells, develop. Differentiated nerve cells called neurons develop from the neuroblasts. Neurons do not divide and are irreplaceable.

15. Glioblasts lead to the formation of glial cells (astrocytes, oligodendrocytes, and microglial cells).

16. During the beginning of the fourth week of gestation, the spinal cord that was derived from the neural tube separates into the ventral basal plate and the dorsal alar plate.

17. The basal plate is considered a motor center, the ventral horn.

18. The alar plate is the sensory center, the dorsal horn in the adult.

19. The cerebellum develops from the mesencephalic vesicle of the neural tube, and the cerebral hemisphere and olfactory bulbs develop from the telencephalon.

CLINICAL NOTES

A number of developmental anomalies result when the nervous system fails to develop appropriately. Congenital malformations of the nervous system occur when the rudimentary structures of the nervous system fail to develop adequately, for example, spina bifida and anencephaly. These anomalies may also be characterized by the absence of cerebral hemispheres, abnormal patterns of sulci and gyri, or absence of several subcortical structures.

Cephalic disorders are congenital conditions caused by abnormal development of the nervous system. They are a major cause of chronic, disabling disorders and sometimes death.

Review Questions

I. Multiple Choice

1. The nervous system develops from the dorsal _____ of the early embryo.
   a. endoderm
   b. ectoderm
   c. mesoderm

2. Nerve cells (neurons and supporting cells) are derived from the outer _____ _____ layer.
   a. mesodermal
   b. ectodermal
   c. endodermal

3. The _____ is noticed in the dorsal midline of the embryo at the sixteenth day of development.
   a. neural plate
   b. neural groove
   c. neither of the above

4. The neural plate changes into a _____ with a _____ along each side.
   a. groove; fold
   b. fold; groove
   c. neither of the above

5. From the neural groove develops the _____ and _____ .
   a. cerebrum; cerebellum
   b. brain; spinal cord
   c. spinal; cranial nerves

6. Neuroectodermal cells that do not participate in forming the neural tube form _____ . These run dorsolaterally along each side of the neural tube.
   a. neural crests
   b. neural troughs
   c. neural processes

7. Dorsal root ganglia of the spinal nerves develop from the _____ .
   a. neural crests
   b. neural plates
   c. neural processes

8. In the rostral portion of the neural tube the _____ develops.
   a. brain
   b. spinal cord
   c. spinal nerves

9. Three primary brain vesicles appear at the end of the _____ week.
   a. fourth
   b. third
   c. second

10. The three primary brain vesicles are the forebrain, midbrain, and _____ .
    a. center brain
    b. hindbrain
    c. lateral brain

11. The secondary brain vesicles are the _____ .
    a. brainstem and cerebellum
    b. cerebrum and cerebellum
    c. brainstem, cerebellum, thalamus, and cerebral hemispheres

12. The _____ within the neural tube develops into the ventricles of the brain and the central canal of the spinal cord.
    a. neural groove
    b. neural canal
    c. neural plate

II. Matching

Match the following abnormalities of the developing nervous system with their appropriate terms.

1. Absence of portions of cerebellum   a. Arachnoid cysts

2. Broader than normal gyri   b. Encephalotrigeminal angiomatosis

3. Cerebrospinal fluid-filled sacs on the arachnoid   c. Agenesis of the cerebellum
   mater

4. Excessive growth of blood vessels on the surface   d. Spina bifida
   of the brain

5. Underdevelopment or complete absence of   e. Neurofibromatoses
   corpus callosum

6. A genetic disorder of the nervous system   f. Macrogyria
   characterized by tumors on the eighth nerve
   that cause skin changes and bone deformities

7. A neural tube defect caused by incomplete   g. Agenesis of the corpus callosum
   development of the brain, spinal cord, and their
   protective coverings, called meninges

III. Matching

Match the following cephalic disorders with their descriptions.

1. Anencephaly

    a. Excessive accumulation of cerebrospinal fluid in the brain

2. Colpocephaly

    b. Neural tube defect that occurs when the cephalic end of the neural tube fails to close, usually between the twenty-third and twenty-sixth days of pregnancy

3. Hydrocephalus

    c. Abnormal enlargement of the occipital horns and lateral ventricles

4. Microcephaly

    d. Failure of development of the embryo's forebrain

5. Holoprosencephaly

    e. Abnormally small head

6. Hydranencephaly

    f. Premature fusion of all sutures

7. Porencephaly

    g. Fusion of coronal suture prematurely

8. Lissencephaly

    h. Larger than average head circumference

9. Schizencephaly

    i. Absence of cerebral hemispheres or replacement of cerebral hemispheres by sacs filled with cerebrospinal fluid

10. Brachycephaly

    j. Cysts or cavities in the cerebral hemispheres

11. Oxycephaly

    k. Microcephaly and lack of convolutions on the cortex

IV. Fill in the Blanks

Provide one-line descriptions for the following terms.

1. Neurulation: _____

2. Neuroectoderm: _____

3. Neural plate: _____

4. Neural folds: _____

5. Neural groove: _____

6. Neural tube: _____

7. Neural crest: _____

8. Neuropore: _____

9. Rhombencephalon: _____

10. Mesencephalon: _____

11. Prosencephalon: _____

12. Myelencephalon: _____

13. Metencephalon: _____

14. Diencephalon: _____

15. Neuroblasts: _____

16. Glioblasts: _____

Answers to Review Questions

I. Multiple Choice

1. b	3. a	5. b	7. a	9. a	11. c
2. b	4. a	6. a	8. a	10. b	12. b

II. Matching

1. c	2. f	3. a	4. b	5. g	6. e	7. d

III Matching

1. b	3. a	5. d	7. j	9. h	11. f
2. c	4. e	6. i	8. k	10. g	

IV. Fill in the Blanks

1. Neurulation: Process of formation of the brain and the spinal cord from the ectoderm during the third week of gestation.

2. Neuroectoderm: Ectoderm from which the neural plate develops.

3. Neural plate: Structure from which the nervous system develops; seen during the third week of embryological development.

4. Neural folds: Identifiable around the neural groove during the third week of gestation when the neural plate transforms into a neural groove along the midline.

5. Neural groove: Tunnel-like structure along the midline, developing during the third week of gestation from the neural plate.

6. Neural tube: Develops during the beginning of the fourth week of gestation from the neural groove; eventually develops into the brain and spinal cord.

7. Neural crest: Segmentally arranged neural tissue surrounding the neural tube; gives rise to spinal ganglia, cranial ganglia, nerve sheaths, and autonomic nerves.

8. Neuropore: Opening at the caudal and rostral ends of the neural tube during the third week of gestation; represents the rudimentary brain and spinal cord.

9. Rhombencephalon: Also called the hindbrain; area that gives rise to future pons, medulla oblongata, and cerebellum.

10. Mesencephalon: Also called the midbrain; houses important structures like the red nucleus, superior colliculi, inferior colliculi, and substantia nigra.

11. Prosencephalon: Also known as the forebrain; area that gives rise to future cerebral hemispheres, ventricles, thalamic nuclei, and other subcallosal structures seen in the medial section of the brain.

12. Myelencephalon: Also known as the future medulla oblongata; develops from rhombencephalon (hindbrain).

13. Metencephalon: Also known as the future pons and cerebellum. Develops from rhombencephalon (hindbrain); the anterior region of the metencephalon develops into the pons whereas the posterior region develops into the cerebellum.

14. Diencephalon: Forms the future ventricles, thalamic nuclei, and other subcallosal structures such as the hypophysis and pineal body.

15. Neuroblasts: Result when, during the fourth week of gestation, the walls of the neural tube thicken; these cells form neurons with primitive axon and dendrites.

16. Glioblasts: Primitive supportive cells seen during the fourth week of gestation in the white matter of the central nervous system; form future astrocytes, oligodendrocytes, and microglia.

Developmental Neurology: Part II

After completing this chapter, the learner will:

- **Be able to describe the continual growth of the brain after birth.**
- **Explain the development of the brain across the life span along with nervous system disorders caused by aging mechanisms.**

Aging of the Nervous System

Age-Related Nervous System Disorders

Clinical Notes

Review Questions

Multiple Choice

Fill in the Blanks

True or False

AGING OF THE NERVOUS SYSTEM

Our nervous system is not spared from aging, which causes irreversible changes. Parkinson's disease and dementia are the two major neurodegenerative disease processes that attack the nervous system.

Unlike most of the body, the brain is not complete at birth. The human brain begins its developmental journey early in prenatal life and continues to develop throughout life. Neural circuits are continuously being modified as the result of new synaptic connections derived from our experiences. Besides synapse formation, myelination is another significant event in postnatal brain development. Cerebral cortex myelination begins in the primary motor and sensory areas and progresses to the association areas that control the more complex integration of perception, thoughts, memories, and feelings. The process of myelination continues until around age 2 years. Myelinated areas are able to transmit neural information.

At birth the brain weighs about 25% of its adult weight. It increases to 75% of adult weight by age 2 years. This weight gain is the result of the proliferation of fibers sent out by neurons. During the first 6 months after birth the subcortical structures (structures below the cortex, e.g., the basal ganglia, cerebellum, and brainstem) develop. The brainstem and cerebellum develop to regulate various vital functions required by the body. By age 1 year the cerebral cortex becomes more active and the infant learns many specialized activities. By the end of the first year, maturation of the auditory pathway takes place. By around age 4 to 5 years the right and left sides of the brain start controlling specific functions. One hemisphere becomes dominant over the other with regard to functions. This is called cerebral asymmetry based on lateralization of functions. For example, spatiotemporal functions are handled by the right hemisphere, while the left brain becomes dominant in language functions. The primary anatomical asymmetry in the brain is found in the left temporal lobe. This may account for the dominance of the left hemisphere in language and cognitive functions. The white fiber tract beneath the temporal lobe is called the planum temporale, which is larger in the left hemisphere.

By age 12 years the brain usually reaches its fully mature weight. The neurons increase in size as dendrites and axons grow to form a dense web of various synapses. The brain apparently shrinks with aging, although estimates on the amount vary. The loss of weight does not indicate the full extent of loss of brain cells, since such cells are replaced by connective tissue and the remaining neurons are often atrophic. Narrowed gyri and deepened sulci are seen in shrunken older brains. Degeneration of various gray matter nuclei also takes place secondary to aging.

AGE-RELATED NERVOUS SYSTEM DISORDERS

Aging is commonly associated with the cognition and physiological performance. Besides heart diseases and cancer, Alzheimer's disease is another cause of death. With aging, total brain weight and volume of the lobes decrease. Atrophy has been noticed in the nuclei responsible for language and memory. Age-associated changes also lead to dilation of ventricles. The age-related changes have been attributed to permanent loss of neurons. Nerve cell mass is lost. Because of atrophy of the brain and spinal cord, weight may decrease significantly from that of the young adult. Atrophy of synapses and tracts and loss of axons are also common. Glial cells also increase with aging because the nervous system is prone to various types of breakdowns.

Functions and release of neurotransmitters also differ in aging populations. Age-related changes in the neurotransmitters are seen in the cortex, hippocampus, thalamus, basal ganglia, and substantia nigra, thus influencing speech, language, and cognition.

CLINICAL NOTES

- Confusion may occur as a result of aging. It is generally characterized by lack of orientation, lack of cohesive thoughts, and inability to make decisions. It may be temporary and reversible. Common causes may relate to head trauma, stroke, concussion, and vitamin deficiency.
- Common nervous system problems in the elderly are delirium, dementia, memory loss caused by aging, and degenerative disorders such as Alzheimer's disease. Delirium involves a rapid alternation between mental states, lack of attention, disorganized thinking, disorientation, changes in sensation and perception, and personality.
- Dementia is a chronic, progressive deterioration of intellect, personality, memory, and communicative function resulting from central nervous system dysfunction (Figure 13-1).
- Dementia may be caused by organic brain syndrome, hydrocephalus, or metabolic causes. Dementia may first be diagnosed when memory impairment becomes apparent. Later, progressive loss of memory, inability to concentrate, confusions, altered sleep patterns, motor system impairment, disorientation, language disturbances, personality changes, etc., characterize the problem.

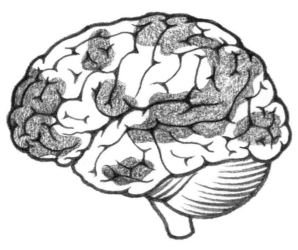

Figure 13-1 Dementia (cortical lesions).

- Another neurodegenerative disease called Creutzfeldt-Jakob disease is usually manifested by mood and personality changes, rapidly progressive dementia, and seizures. This progression to dementia is much faster. Lesions encompass six layers of the cortex.
- In corticobasal degeneration, progressive aphasia is seen usually with lesions in the left frontal lobe. Neurons show swollen cytoplasm and loss of Nissl's granules in the cytoplasm. A combination of motor and cognitive deficits is seen.
- The main characteristic of Alzheimer's disease is dementia. It is a progressive disease characterized by prominent language degeneration and cognitive deficits. Neuritic plaques and neurofibrillary tangles are found throughout the brain.
- Frontal lobe dementia is a progressive disorder caused by a lesion in the frontal lobe. Personality changes rather than cognitive or memory loss characterize the disorder. Dysarthria, orofacial apraxia, and widespread cognitive deficits are seen.
- Pick's desease is characterized by prominent language deterioration accompanied by dementia. Presenile onset, personality change, disinhibition, reduced speech fluency, and verbal stereotypes are typical. The neuropathology of Pick's disease involves a focal lobar atrophy affecting the frontal and temporal lobes of one or both hemispheres. Cortical neurons evidence "Pick bodies," which are large cytoplasmic inclusions. Parietal lobe atrophy may also accompany this disorder.
- Idiopathic Parkinson's disease is seen in many aging individuals. It results from loss of nerve cells from the central nervous system. Neurons of the substantia nigra, basal ganglia, and brainstem degenerate (Figure 13-2). Because of a loss of neurons in the substantia nigra, a deficiency in dopamine, a neurotransmitter, results. Three main features of this disease are tremor at rest, rigidity, and bradykinesia (slowness of movement).
- Transient global amnesia is a syndrome that tends to occur in patients over age 50 years. It involves a temporary and selective memory loss for a few hours. During the period of amnesia, the patient cannot remember recent events and does not retain any new information. Its pathological mechanism remains unclear.

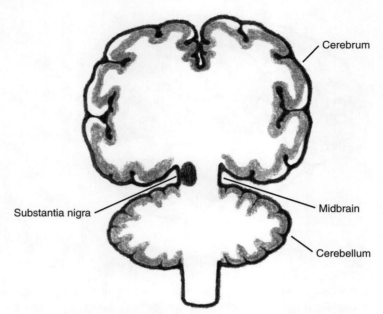

Figure 13-2   Parkinson's disease (damage in substantia nigra).

Review Questions

I. Multiple Choice

1. Loss of gray matter results from _____ .
   a. disintegration of the myelin sheath
   b. breakdown of synapses
   c. axonal degeneration
   d. none of the above

2. Loss of white matter results from _____ .
   a. death of cell bodies
   b. axonal degeneration
   c. degeneration of the myelin sheath
   d. a and c

3. Neurons alter their neural transmission mechanisms with age, which directly affects

   _____ and the release of various neurotransmitters.
   a. action potentials
   b. resting potentials
   c. membrane potentials

4. Aging of the nervous system causes changes in _____ .
   a. emotional behavior and personality
   b. muscle activities
   c. motor coordination
   d. all of the above

5. Parkinson's disease, an age-related disease of the nervous system, occurs because of

   _____ .

   a. degeneration of the medulla oblongata
   b. increase of dopamine levels
   c. degeneration of the substantia nigra
   d. degeneration of the frontal lobe
   e. none of the above

6. Alzheimer's disease, an age-related disease of the nervous system, is characterized by

   _____ .

   a. progressive loss of intellectual functions
   b. memory impairments
   c. behavioral and personality changes
   d. all of the above

7. In Alzheimer's disease, neuronal loss in the _____ and _____ _____ are seen.
   a. hippocampus; cerebral cortex
   b. thalamus; pons
   c. midbrain; spinal cord
   d. epithalamus; subthalamus

8. Because of aging, myopathic and degenerative changes develop in response to _____ _____ .
   a. reduction of conduction velocities
   b. loss of motor neurons
   c. reduction of muscle weight
   d. a and b
   e. all of the above

9. Aging of the nervous system increases susceptibility to _____ .
   a. extra growth of tissues
   b. infections
   c. vascular diseases
   d. b and c
   e. all of the above

10. Findings in patients with Alzheimer's disease include _____ .
    a. significant neuronal loss
    b. loss of dendrites
    c. neurofibrillary tangles and plaques
    d. all of the above

11. Aging has a positive effect on the deterioration of language performance in all areas except _____ .
    a. semantics/vocabulary
    b. syntax/grammar
    c. phonology/sound system of language
    d. pragmatics/use of language in various situations

12. Pick's disease is a cortical dementing disease characterized by _____ .
    a. severe cell loss
    b. atrophy in the frontal and temporal lobes
    c. atrophy in the occipital lobe
    d. a and b

13. In _____ dementia, personality changes, rather than cognitive or memory loss, predominate the clinical picture.
    a. Alzheimer's
    b. frontal lobe
    c. parietal lobe
    d. none of the above
    e. all of the above

14. In the early stages of Alzheimer's disease, _____ impairment appears to be the only major cognitive deficit.
    a. speech
    b. memory
    c. language
    d. attention

15. In the middle stages of Alzheimer's disease, behavioral and _____ changes become more evident.
    a. speech
    b. language
    c. personality
    d. none of the above

16. In the late stages of Alzheimer's disease, _____ are seen.
    a. profound cognitive changes
    b. depression
    c. appearance changes
    d. all of the above

II. Fill in the Blanks

Determine whether the following causes of dementia are reversible or irreversible.

1. Alzheimer's disease: _____

2. Pick's disease: _____

3. Tumors of the brain: _____

4. Renal failure: _____

5. Thyroid disease: _____

6. Parkinson's disease: _____

7. Hypoglycemia: _____

8. Vitamin deficiency: _____

9. Congestive heart failure: _____

10. Huntington's disease: _____

III. True or False

1. The dementia of mild Alzheimer's disease patients is likely to be confused with the effects of normal aging on cognition.
2. The dementia associated with mild Pick's disease is nonprogressive.
3. Mental changes are not associated with vascular diseases.

4. Aging usually does not affect language, memory, and intellect.
5. Decline in discourse comprehension and generative naming is usually seen with aging.
6. Rapid forgetting is the primary problem with mild dementia.
7. Depression is not very common in the elderly.
8. Nonfluent speech and muteness are most commonly seen in Pick's disease.
9. Vascular dementia may exist without a history of hypertension.
10. Lewy body dementia patients experience fluctuating cognitive impairments.
11. In addition to Lewy bodies, neuritic plaques and neurofibrillary tangles may be present in patients with Lewy body dementia.
12. Evidence of subcortical dysfunction may be seen in patients diagnosed with vascular dementia.
13. Pseudobulbar palsy may exist in vascular dementia.
14. Occipital lobe degeneration is seen in Pick's disease.
15. Progressive aphasia is a degenerative cortical disease.
16. The onset of Alzheimer's disease is characterized by episodic memory problems.
17. In advanced stages of dementia, patients experience global intellectual deterioration.
18. Psychiatric symptoms do not exist in Alzheimer's disease.

Answers to Review Questions

I. Multiple Choice

1. d	3. a	5. c	7. a	9. e	11. c	13. b	15. c
2. d	4. d	6. d	8. e	10. d	12. d	14. b	16. d

II. Fill in the Blanks

1. Irreversible

2. Reversible

3. Reversible

4. Irreversible

5. Reversible

6. Irreversible

7. Reversible

8. Reversible

9. Irreversible

10. Irreversible

III. True or False

1. True	4. False	7. False	10. True	13. True	16. True
2. False	5. True	8. True	11. True	14. False	17. True
3. False	6. True	9. False	12. True	15. True	18. False

14

Case Studies: Pediatric Neurogenic Communication Disorders

OUTLINE

Case Studies and Review Questions

Developmental neuropathology is a complex field. The case studies presented in this chapter are designed to help decipher the complex neuroanatomical correlates, behaviors, and pathological factors operating in various pediatric neurological conditions.

Case Studies and Review Questions

A 4-year-old girl with a history of chronic otitis media is evaluated for "short stature" evidenced by a gradual decrease in height percentile from 20% (at birth) to < 3% (at age 4 years). The physical examination is remarkable only for slight backward rotation of the ears and small mandible (micrognathia). X-ray studies demonstrate delayed bone maturation.

1. What is the possible diagnosis?
   a. Turner's syndrome
   b. Treacher-Collins syndrome
   c. Down's syndrome

2. What type of chromosomal abnormality causes short stature, dysmorphic abnormalities, hearing loss, and other dysgenesis?
   a. missing or absent Y chromosome
   b. missing or absent X chromosome

A 5-year-old child has headaches, progressive ataxia, and hydrocephalus. The diagnostic work-up (magnetic resonance imaging [MRI] and computed tomography [CT] scan) reveal a mass in the posterior fossa.

1. The mass is most likely to be a tumor in the _____ .
   a. cerebrum
   b. cerebellum
   c. brainstem

2. The most common types of tumors in children are infratentorial tumors.
   a. true
   b. false

A 3-year-old child comes to the clinic with a history of trauma during birth; a neurological examination revealed severe contractures, increased reflexes, and microcephaly. The child is unable to control movements in her limbs. She has both speech and feeding problems.

1. What is the possible diagnosis?
   a. cerebral palsy
   b. stroke
   c. autism

2. The possible lesion is in the _____ .
   a. cerebellum
   b. pyramidal tract
   c. brainstem

CASE STUDY IV

A 4-year-old boy comes to the clinic, and his parents state that the child has had repeated seizures occurring several times a day.

1. What is the diagnosis?
   a. epilepsy
   b. stroke
   c. paralysis

2. What is the possible cause of these seizures?
   a. unusual and strong bursts of electrical energy in the brain
   b. loss of astrocytes
   c. loss of glial cells

CASE STUDY V

A female infant was born to a mother who smoked heavily during pregnancy. The infant had a laryngeal web and showed delayed motor development. MRI results suggested delayed myelination patterns. At age 4 years the child has mildly coarse facial features with a prominent mandible and a simple philtrum. Excessive movements in the limbs are noted. A broad-based, stiff, and jerky gait is also seen. Distortion of chromosome 15 is found.

1. What is the possible diagnosis?
   a. Down's syndrome
   b. Treacher-Collins syndrome
   c. Angelman syndrome

2. A laryngeal web interferes with _____ .
   a. breathing
   b. voice
   c. both of the above

3. Delayed myelination patterns suggest an overall developmental delay.
   a. true
   b. false

4. A prominent mandible indicates a _____ malocclusion.
   a. Class II
   b. Class III

5. Excessive movements in the limbs may result from _____ .
   a. damage in the pyramidal system
   b. damage in the extrapyramidal system

CASE STUDY VI

A 2-year-old child comes to you with paralysis of both upper and one lower extremity.

1. What is the diagnosis?
   a. diplegia
   b. triplegia
   c. quadriplegia

2. Presence or absence of primitive reflexes helps us diagnose neurological disorders.
   a. true
   b. false

CASE STUDY VII

A 6½ -year-old girl comes to the clinic with a history of mental retardation and seizure disorders. She has numerous light brown areas usually located over the trunk. She also has scoliosis.

1. What is the possible diagnosis?
   a. neurofibromatosis
   b. cerebellar tumors
   c. brainstem tumors

2. What is the most important characteristic of this disease?
   a. lesions of the vascular system and the viscera
   b. cutaneous pigmentation
   c. multiple tumors within the central and peripheral nervous systems

CASE STUDY VIII

A 5-year-old boy comes to the clinic with delayed onset of speech. He is hyperactive and clumsy and has large ears. Neurological examination documents the presence of impaired fine motor coordination and a short attention span. Genetic analysis indicates chromosomal abnormality linked with the X chromosome.

1. What is the syndrome called?
   a. absent-X syndrome
   b. fragile-X syndrome
   c. Turner's syndrome

2. What are the behavioral manifestations of this syndrome?
   a. attention deficit disorder
   b. mental retardation
   c. developmental expressive aphasia
   d. all of the above

CASE STUDY IX

A 4-year-old boy comes to the clinic with a history of weakness of the hip and shoulder girdles. He has gait disturbances and difficulties with physical activities such as climbing stairs and jumping. The child is also mentally retarded.

1. What is the possible diagnosis?
   a. juvenile form of myasthenia gravis
   b. poliomyelitis
   c. Duchenne muscular dystrophy

2. This disease is transmitted as an X-linked recessive trait and therefore affects _____

   _____ .
   a. only males
   b. only females
   c. both males and females

3. What is the course of this disease?
   a. nonprogressive
   b. progressive

CASE STUDY X

A 5-year-old child comes to the clinic with complaints of fever, headaches, and vomiting. The parents complain that the child is very inactive and lethargic. The child has sleep disturbances and exhibits temperaments that are difficult to control.

1. What is the possible diagnosis?
   a. measles
   b. rubella
   c. encephalitis

2. Meningitis may also be involved in this condition.
   a. true
   b. false

3. The child with this condition may also exhibit focal neurological signs such as _____

   _____ .
   a. aphasia
   b. ataxia
   c. cranial nerve palsies
   d. all of the above

4. Sequelae of the above condition include _____ .
   a. personality problems
   b. seizures
   c. spasticity
   d. all of the above

CASE STUDY XI

A 6-year-old child comes with a complaint of headache, vomiting, and specific neurological signs (unsteady gait, slow and slurred speech, and motor incoordination).

1. What is the possible diagnosis?
   a. cerebellar tumor
   b. tumor of the fourth ventricle
   c. a and b

2. Increased intracranial pressure gives rise to headache and vomiting.
   a. true
   b. false

3. Early symptoms of these tumors may also include _____ .
   a. academic deficits
   b. motor deficits
   c. Anorexia and weight loss

4. Diadochokinetic rate of the child's speech will be _____.
   a. fast
   b. slow

CASE STUDY XII

A child is seen for abnormally small head (less than two standard deviations below the mean for age and gender). The child has normal face size and folded scalp.

1. This condition is called _____ ; it results from metabolic disorders.
   a. megalencephaly
   b. micrencephaly
   c. holoprosencephaly

2. If it were found that the two hemispheres have failed to develop and as a result a large fluid-filled cavity results, what would this condition be called?
   a. anencephaly
   b. holoprosencephaly
   c. micrencephaly

3. In this latter case, does the interhemispheric pressure increase?
   a. yes
   b. no

4. What is the possible cause?
   a. radiation problems
   b. metabolic disorders

CASE STUDY XIII

A female infant one day after birth has feeble cry and movements. She is unable to suck and swallow, and her breathing pattern is shallow and impaired. Muscular weakness and hypotonia are generalized.

1. What is the possible diagnosis?
   a. metabolic myopathy
   b. muscular dystrophy
   c. myasthenia gravis

2. Which characteristic/s is(are) true about this disorder?
   a. possible recovery after rest
   b. absence of Moro and deep tendon reflexes
   c. undue weakness and fatigue after the contraction of voluntary muscles

3. This disease occasionally runs in families.
   a. true
   b. false

CASE STUDY XIV

A 12-month-old infant is brought to the clinic because of poor feeding, vomiting, fever, and drowsiness over the course of 3 days. The parents report convulsions and stiffness of the neck.

1. What is the possible diagnosis?
   a. epilepsy
   b. meningitis

2. The examination will show that the child has _____ .
   a. fever and drowsiness
   b. weakness of the eye muscles and face
   c. neck rigidity

3. As the infection progresses, the patient might become _____ .
   a. less responsive, confused, and eventually comatose
   b. hyperactive
   c. psychotic

4. Neurological examination may reveal evidence of cranial nerve palsies. Which cranial nerves will be damaged?
   a. VI
   b. VII
   c. VIII
   d. all of the above

CASE STUDY XV

A developmentally delayed boy age 5 years is hospitalized for sudden hearing loss because of an infection. Sequelae of the disease include a stroke and seizure disorders that have left the boy with delayed speech milestones. An audiological evaluation shows profound sensorineural hearing loss in both ears.

1. What is the possible diagnosis?
    a. meningitis
    b. otitis media
    c. otosclerosis

2. This disease is characterized by _____ .
    a. inflammation of the membranes of the brain and spinal cord
    b. ischemic attacks
    c. metabolic disorders

CASE STUDY XVI

A 9-year-old boy is referred to the clinic with a history of mental retardation and delayed speech and language development. He demonstrates a progressive sensorineural hearing loss in the high frequencies. DNA analysis indicates a mitochondrial disease.

1. What is the consequence of this type of disease?
    a. breakdown of synapses of auditory neurons
    b. shearing of the tympanic membrane
    c. disruption of synchronous firing of individual neurons

2. Major types of disorders related to mitochondrial encephalomyopathy include all of the following except _____ .
    a. ophthalmoplegia
    b. myoclonus epilepsy
    c. stroke-like episodes
    d. atrophy

CASE STUDY XVII

A 2-day-old infant comes to the clinic with an open spine. The spinal cord and its protective coverings are protruding from an opening in the spine. The infant's head is noticeably large.

1. What is the possible diagnosis?
    a. myelomeningocele
    b. spinal dislocation
    c. meningocele

2. Why is the infant's head so large?
    a. The infant has macrocephaly because of the lack of decay of neurons.
    b. The infant has hydrocephalus, which is often associated with this condition.
    c. The infant has a learning disability.

3. What is the cause of this disorder?
   a. It is a neural tube defect that involves incomplete development of the brain, spinal cord, and/or their protective coverings.
   b. It is an autosomal recessive disorder.
   c. It is caused by perinatal trauma.

CASE STUDY XVIII

A 6-year-old girl comes to the clinic with complaints of recurrent vomiting, irritability, combativeness, disorientation, confusion, delirium, convulsions, and loss of consciousness at times. These symptoms followed an episode of flu. On physical examination the child's liver and other vital organs show fatty deposits.

1. What is the possible diagnosis?
   a. Reye's syndrome
   b. meningitis
   c. encephalitis
   d. carbon monoxide poisoning

2. Increased intracranial pressure is noted due to _____ .
   a. coma
   b. seizures
   c. cerebral edema

CASE STUDY XIX

A floppy 18-month-old child is seen in the clinic with purposeless flailing and writhing movements of the hands. She avoids eye contact and does not like to be cuddled. No babbling or vocalization is noticed. The parents report seizures occurring at least three times in a week.

1. What is the possible diagnosis?
   a. Reye's syndrome
   b. Rett's syndrome
   c. lead poisoning

2. What are the consequences of Rett's syndrome?
   a. loss of motor skills
   b. awkward gait and trunk movements
   c. mental retardation
   d. language disturbances
   e. all of the above

Answers to Review Questions

Case Study I
1. a   2. b

Case Study II
1. b   2. a

Case Study III
1. a   2. b

Case Study IV
1. a   2. a

Case Study V
1. c   2. c   3. a   4. b   5. b

Case Study VI
1. b   2. a

Case Study VII
1. a   2. c

Case Study VIII
1. b   2. d

Case Study IX
1. c   2. c   3. b

Case Study X
1. c   2. a   3. d   4. d

Case Study XI

1. a 2. a 3. b 4. b

Case Study XII

1. b 2. b 3. a 4. a

Case Study XIII

1. b 2. c 3. a

Case Study XIV

1. b 2. c 3. a 4. d

Case Study XV

1. a 2. a

Case Study XVI

1. a 2. d

Case Study XVII

1. a 2. b 3. a

Case Study XVIII

1. a 2. c

Case Study XIX

1. b 2. e

15

Case Studies: Adult Neurogenic Communication Disorders

OUTLINE

Case Studies and Review Questions

This chapter focuses on adult case studies of neurological conditions. Each case study has been selected to represent one of the well-known neurological disorders of communication.

Case Studies and Review Questions

A 40-year-old man comes to the clinic with unintelligible speech characterized by strained voice, hypernasality, slow speech, and weak voice. On examination, tongue atrophy and fasciculations of the tongue and face are seen. The patient is unable to communicate well and is emotionally labile.

1. What is the possible diagnosis?
   a. amyotrophic lateral sclerosis
   b. multiple sclerosis
   c. myasthenia gravis

2. An individual with this diagnosis typically manifests all of the following except _____ .
   a. fasciculations
   b. muscle weakness
   c. sensory loss
   d. dementia
   e. muscle atrophy

3. Which of the following elements does not belong to this motor neuron disease?
   a. degeneration of motor nuclei of the midbrain, pons, and medulla
   b. degeneration of the frontal lobe and pyramidal tracts
   c. degeneration of the anterior horn cells of the spinal cord
   d. degeneration of the posterior horn cells of the spinal cord

4. Electromyography will show typical _____ .
   a. denervation patterns with fibrillation potentials
   b. decrease in nerve conduction velocities
   c. increase of motor unit action potentials
   d. all of the above

5. Alternate motion rate of articulators is usually _____ .
   a. fast
   b. slow

6. What type of dysarthria will be manifested in this disease?
   a. mixed
   b. LMN
   c. UMN

7. Which one does not belong to characteristics of UMN lesions?
   a. no wasting/atrophy
   b. increased tone
   c. increased reflexes and clonus
   d. fasciculations

8. Which are characteristics of LMN lesions?
   a. wasting
   b. weakness
   c. decreased reflexes
   d. all of the above
   e. none of the above

9. _____ is the ultimate cause of death in this disease.
   a. Drooling
   b. Dysphagia
   c. Respiratory insufficiency

CASE STUDY II

A 67-year-old woman demonstrates rigidity in all limbs and gait disturbances. She is slow to initiate limb movements and walks with short shuffling steps. She has a masklike facies and shows tremors of the head, lower extremities, and upper extremities during rest. She also reports depression. Marked spasticity is noticed in her arms.

1. What is the possible diagnosis?
   a. myasthenia gravis
   b. amyotrophic lateral sclerosis
   c. Parkinson's disease

2. What is the possible pathophysiology of the disease?
   a. degeneration of the cerebral cortex
   b. demyelination of nerve cells
   c. degeneration of the substantia nigra and other basal ganglion structures

3. What type of dysarthria will you expect in this patient?
   a. hypokinetic
   b. hyperkinetic
   c. flaccid

4. What type of tremor is usually seen in this disease?
   a. tremors at rest
   b. tremors during action

5. Is resting tremor a characteristic of benign essential tremor too?
   a. yes
   b. no

CASE STUDY III

A 56-year-old man came for care of pure motor hemiplegia affecting the face, arm, and leg as a result of infarction in the internal capsule or in the basis pons. There is no evidence of aphasia, visuospatial neglect, agnosia, or apraxia. During a follow-up visit, it is noted that the patient has recovered very well and is quite functional in everyday activities.

1. What is the possible diagnosis?
   a. lacunar stroke
   b. irreversible transient ischemic attack

2. Pure sensory stroke is another possible diagnosis fitting the clinical picture. It is caused by

   small infarcts in the _____ .
   a. thalamus
   b. basal ganglia

CASE STUDY IV

A 50-year-old woman with a history of hypertension reports sudden onset of blindness, swallowing difficulties, and slurred speech. After 22 hours, she is able to regain all the functions she had lost.

1. What is the possible diagnosis?
   a. irreversible transient ischemic attack
   b. reversible transient ischemic attack

2. What is the possible cause of this episode?
   a. permanent neuronal damage
   b. temporary interruption of blood supply

3. If the middle cerebral artery is occluded, what types of symptoms will be seen?
   a. dysphasia
   b. dyslexia
   c. dysgraphia
   d. all of the above

4. If the vertebrobasilar territory is disturbed, the following symptoms may be noted.
   a. diplopia
   b. vertigo
   c. motor and sensory loss
   d. none of the above
   e. all of the above

5. An MRI scan will be able to detect _____ .
   a. cerebral herniation
   b. brainstem infarction
   c. small deep hemispheric infarcts
   d. all of the above

6. Which statement(s) best explain(s) the pathophysiology of stroke?
   a. occlusion of the artery because of thrombosis or embolus
   b. lack of collateral blood supply
   c. infarction of the central nervous system structures
   d. all of the above

CASE STUDY V

A 25-year-old man is admitted to the hospital after a minor head-on collision. He did not lose consciousness but is not able to answer questions in the examination room because he is confused and this problem persists even after 8 hours. The patient exhibits rhinorrhea, otorrhea, and orbital hematoma.

1. What is the possible underlying cause of the confusion?
   a. brain injury resulting from skull fracture
   b. penetrating injury
   c. coma

2. Will the patient retain normal mood, behavior, and communication?
   a. yes
   b. no

CASE STUDY VI

HT is a 90-year-old man who suffered a stroke recently. He has lost his ability to comprehend simple language. Jargon, neologisms, and paraphasias characterize his speech. Repetition is very poor. He appears to be highly confused and disoriented.

1. What is the possible diagnosis?
   a. global aphasia
   b. conduction aphasia
   c. Wernicke's aphasia

2. What is the possible site of the lesion?
   a. arcuate fasciculus
   b. anterior and posterior perisylvian area
   c. posterior perisylvian area

3. What is the possible prognosis?
   a. fair
   b. poor

CASE STUDY VII

MC is a 39-year-old right-handed man who exhibits severe nonfluent and agrammatic speech after a left-hemisphere stroke. However, MC is able to comprehend speech.

1. What is the diagnosis?
   a. Broca's aphasia
   b. transcortical sensory aphasia
   c. global aphasia

2. The CT scan is likely to show a lesion in the ————————— .
   a. parietal lobe
   b. limbic lobe
   c. frontotemporal lobe

3. Which factor(s) is(are) likely to indicate a good prognosis?
   a. comprehension abilities
   b. no associated problems
   c. age
   d. all of the above

CASE STUDY VIII

Mr. WS was a 50-year-old man who was involved in a road accident 1 month ago. He had been suffering from a closed head injury since that time. Initially he was not able to respond to any type of stimulus, but then he began showing signs of cognitive dysfunction and became nonambulatory. He died as the result of a massive internal hemorrhage.

1. Which of the following diagnoses best suits this clinical situation?
   a. stroke
   b. TBI

2. Is it likely that the meninges were intact after the accident?
   a. yes
   b. no

3. What possible dysfunctions would be seen in this patient while living?
   a. memory deficits
   b. language problems
   c. alertness and attention problems
   d. all of the above

4. Why did the patient become nonambulatory?
   a. because of severe quadriplegic conditions
   b. because of lack of environmental control
   c. because of reduced sensory stimulation

5. Which test would you use to measure the level of consciousness while the patient is in a coma?
   a. test of discourse processing
   b. Glasgow Coma Scale
   c. Western Aphasia Battery
   d. none of the above

CASE STUDY IX

KO is a 45-year-old woman who had a stroke 3 months ago. She has been showing very good signs of recovery regarding speech and other motor functions. Nonfluent utterances, intact comprehension, and intact repetition characterize her speech.

1. What is the possible diagnosis?
   a. anomic aphasia
   b. Broca's aphasia
   c. global aphasia
   d. none of the above

2. Is it likely that writing is impaired?
   a. yes
   b. no

3. Will naming be impaired?
   a. yes
   b. no

4. Will the patient show paraphasias?
   a. yes
   b. no

CASE STUDY X

Mrs. Y suffered both cortical and subcortical strokes within the last few months. Family members have started noticing confusions, paranoid behaviors, intellectual deteriorations, and disorientations.

1. What is the diagnosis?
   a. multi-infarct aphasia
   b. multi-infarct dementia
   c. multi-infarct corticobasal damage

2. Will the patient show memory problems?
   a. yes
   b. no

3. A CT scan could show which of the following?
   a. damage in the gray and white matter of the brain
   b. damage in the cell bodies
   c. damage in the cerebellum

4. What is the usual prognosis in this condition?
   a. good
   b. poor

5. Will the patient show impaired judgment and impaired abstract thinking?
   a. yes
   b. no

6. Which one of the following is a reversible cause of dementia?
   a. nutritional disorders
   b. Pick's disease
   c. Parkinson's disease

CASE STUDY XI

SA is a 62-year-old man having reduced tactile and spatial sensation, apraxia, visual field deficits, and dyslexia because of a tumor. He also has seizure disorders. Surgery will be done as soon as a neuroradiological examination is completed.

1. Where is the tumor located?
   a. frontal lobe
   b. temporal lobe
   c. parietal lobe
   d. occipital lobe

2. What might be the possible finding on MRI?
   a. displacement of cerebral tissue in the cranium
   b. edema
   c. both

3. SA's seizures are not localized anymore. What kind of seizure is he now experiencing?
   a. generalized
   b. partial
   c. neither of the above

4. What is the prognosis?
   a. poor
   b. good

CASE STUDY XII

SD is a 23-year-old woman who has organic voice tremor and myoclonus.

1. What kind of dysarthria is she likely to evidence?
   a. hyperkinetic
   b. ataxic

2. What would be the type of voice quality?
   a. strained
   b. weak voice
   c. neither of the above

3. Where is the lesion most likely located?
   a. extrapyramidal tract
   b. cerebellum

4. Would this client benefit from voice therapy?
   a. yes
   b. no

CASE STUDY XIII

SF is a 45-year-old man who suffered a hemorrhage recently. He exhibits fluent paraphasias, intact repetition, and poor comprehension.

1. What is most likely the best diagnosis?
   a. Broca's aphasia
   b. conduction aphasia
   c. Wernicke's aphasia

2. What is the possible site of lesion?
   a. arcuate fasciculus
   b. frontal lobe
   c. occipital lobe

3. Will naming be impaired?
   a. yes
   b. no

CASE STUDY XIV

A 21-year-old man complains of headache that has been present for 1 month and a recent onset of seizures. He shows severe intellectual decline and attention deficits.

1. Where is the possible site of lesion?
   a. temporal lobe
   b. occipital lobe
   c. parietal lobe
   d. frontal lobe

2. What is the type of lesion?
   a. hemorrhage
   b. thrombosis
   c. tumor

3. What will happen if the left lateral ventricle is compressed due to the lesion?
   a. intracranial pressure increases
   b. CSF increases
   c. no effect

CASE STUDY XV

DS is a 56-year-old man with a history of severe hypertension. He has good comprehension, but word-finding pauses and circumlocutions characterize his verbal output.

1. What is the possible diagnosis?
   a. transcortical aphasia
   b. Wernicke's aphasia
   c. anomic aphasia

2. Where is the possible site of lesion?
   a. left temporal gyrus
   b. left angular gyrus
   c. both of the above

3. Will reading be intact?
   a. yes
   b. no

CASE STUDY XVI

DF is an 86-year-old woman with a history of aneurysms. Recently she suffered a massive stroke and was in a coma for 8 days. Since recovery, she has been living in a vegetative state with no speech at all.

1. What is the diagnosis?
   a. moderate Broca's aphasia
   b. severe Wernicke's aphasia
   c. severe global aphasia

2. Where is the site of lesion?
   a. nondominant frontotemporal area
   b. right hemispheric area
   c. left frontotemporoparietal area

3. What will be one of the associated signs?
   a. hemiparesis
   b. hemiplegia
   c. both of the above

CASE STUDY XVII

SE is a 35-year-old man who is complaining of a vision problem and then nystagmus. He is also experiencing weakness and numbness of the arms. He shows ataxia of speech accompanied by tremors. Neurophysiological examinations indicate replacement of myelin by glial tissues.

1. What is the possible diagnosis?
   a. myasthenia gravis
   b. Wilson's disease
   c. multiple sclerosis

2. Where might the lesions be located?
   a. PNS
   b. CNS
   c. both of the above

3. What would an MRI scan reveal?
   a. diffuse lesions in the cerebral hemispheres
   b. lesion in the occipital lobe
   c. multiple degenerative plaques in the white matter of the cerebral hemispheres

4. Is this problem progressive?
   a. yes
   b. no

CASE STUDY XVIII

SD is a 46-year-old man with a history of seizures. Recently he has started noticing apraxia, dyslexia, and dysgraphia. CT scan indicates a mass in one of his lobes.

1. Where is the site of lesion?
   a. temporal lobe
   b. occipital lobe
   c. parietal lobe

2. Will SD evidence visual field defects?
   a. yes
   b. no

CASE STUDY XIX

SC is a 50-year-old woman with swallowing and speech problems. She reports aspiration and nasal regurgitation during food intake. Her speech is flaccid dysarthric. A neurological examination indicates fasciculations and muscular weakness resulting from abnormal neurotransmitters.

1. What is the possible diagnosis?
   a. ALS
   b. Parkinson's disease
   c. myasthenia gravis

2. Will you be able to record normal muscular contractions using an EMG?
   a. yes
   b. no

3. Are the respiratory muscles also affected?
   a. yes
   b. no

CASE STUDY XX

A 36-year-old woman comes to the clinic with a complaint of fatigue. She reports becoming tired after short walks. She also complains that her speech becomes slurred after speaking for about an hour.

1. What is the possible diagnosis?
   a. multiple sclerosis
   b. Pick's disease
   c. myasthenia gravis

2. What is the cause of this disease?
   a. insufficient production of receptor proteins at the neuromuscular junctions
   b. degeneration of the cortex
   c. degeneration of sensory neurons

3. Identify the group of signs and symptoms related to this disorder.
   a. absent plantar responses, multiple tumors, and vertigo
   b. ptosis, dysarthria, and dysphagia

4. Would you see any sign of fasciculation and atrophy?
   a. yes
   b. no

CASE STUDY XXI

A 65-year-old man is complaining of word-finding difficulties and having increasing speech difficulties. He is very fluent, has minor spelling errors, and cannot concentrate well on reading tasks. He has very good orientation, memory, and judgment abilities. He does not show any signs of paralysis or paresis.

1. What is the possible diagnosis?
   a. Parkinson's disease
   b. primary progressive aphasia
   c. Wernicke's aphasia

2. What will a neurological evaluation typically show?
   a. degeneration of the frontal lobe
   b. temporal lobe atrophy
   c. lesion in the parietal lobe

3. Does this neurological disorder have a good long-term prognosis?
   a. yes
   b. no

4. In considering differential diagnoses between various neurological disorders for the above diagnosis, which group of disorders should be considered?
   a. dementia, delirium, and multi-infarct dementia
   b. Wernicke's aphasia and Huntington's chorea
   c. anomia and Wernicke's aphasia

CASE STUDY XXII

A 31-year-old German-English soldier received a gunshot wound in the left cerebral hemisphere; as a consequence he became completely aphasic. He learned English when he was 28 years old. He could not express himself orally or in writing. He was also unable to understand spoken or written languages. During the period of spontaneous recovery while he was left in a nursing home in New York, he was observed to understand written English words. He returned to Germany after 6 months. Slowly he began to speak, read, and write in German, demonstrating no repetition or expression of English words, although he retained the ability to comprehend simple functional English vocabulary words.

1. Why was spontaneous recovery seen in English and not in German initially even though German was the first language of the soldier?
   a. English language was probably localized in the right hemisphere.
   b. English language was recovered because of the sociolinguistic setting in the nursing home.
   c. German is comparatively more difficult than English.

2. In this case, spontaneous recovery was significant because the patient was _____

   _____ .
   a. bilingual
   b. young

3. In recovery from aphasia, a foreign language may show pre-eminence over the native tongue if the patient was using this foreign language when he becomes aphasic. Is this statement supported by observed behavior?
   a. yes
   b. no

4. Does the recovery pattern for this patient follow Pitre's rule that states, in aphasia the language that was used most frequently is generally the last to be lost or the first to return?
   a. yes
   b. no

5. Does this case study follow Ribot's law, which states that languages acquired earlier in life are easier to retain longer in polyglot aphasics?
   a. yes
   b. no

6. While looking at the recovery patterns of polyglot aphasics, the linguistic surroundings of the patient and the verbal stimulation he or she receives from the environment may influence language restoration to a considerable extent.
   a. true
   b. false

CASE STUDY XXIII

A 70-year-old woman suffered a severe cerebral trauma in a car accident that has left her without speech. Neurological examination shows no aphasia, apraxia, or cognitive-linguistic dysfunction. Her voice is hypernasal and hoarse.

1. What could be the reason of speechlessness?
   a. severe sensory deficits
   b. severe motor deficits
   c. cognitive deficits

2. What would a neuroradiologic diagnostic report reveal?
   a. frontal lobe lesions
   b. temporal lobe lesions
   c. parietal lobe lesions

CASE STUDY XXIV

A patient came to the clinic with a chronic right hemisphere ischemic stroke.

1. What kind of symptoms is he likely to show?
   a. left hemiplegia
   b. language processing problems at higher levels
   c. hemisensory deficits
   d. none of the above
   e. all of the above

2. Will the patient demonstrate personality and behavioral changes?
   a. yes
   b. no

CASE STUDY XXV

A 46-year-old man presents with a generalized choreiform disorder that began at age 43 years. He has dysarthria of speech. His mother died as the result of an unknown psychotic disorder.

1. What is the possible diagnosis?
   a. Huntington's disease
   b. Parkinson's disease
   c. Wilson's disease

2. Is this disorder an autosomal dominant disorder?
   a. yes
   b. no

CASE STUDY XXVI

A 50-year-old woman is brought to the clinic for a neurological evaluation. She is diagnosed with a sleep disorder and paranoid behaviors. She is taking neuroleptic drugs. The patient has repetitive, voluntary, purposeless movements. Facial grimacing, tongue protrusion, lip smacking, puckering, pursing, and rapid eye blinking are quite common.

1. What is the possible diagnosis?
   a. Huntington's chorea
   b. tardive dyskinesia
   c. Sydenham's chorea

2. Dyskinesia refers to _____ .
   a. defective rhythm
   b. atonia in the muscles
   c. difficulty in performing voluntary movements due to presence of involuntary movements

CASE STUDY XXVII

In the following diagrams, identify the pathological conditions based on the shaded areas of the cortex.

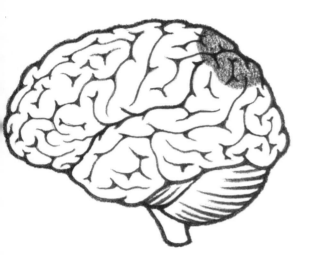

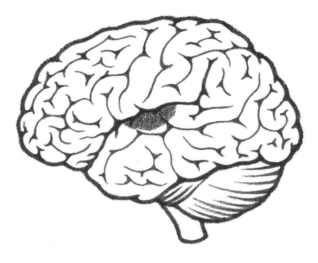

1. _____

2. _____

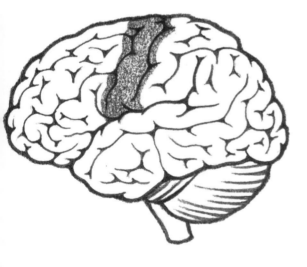

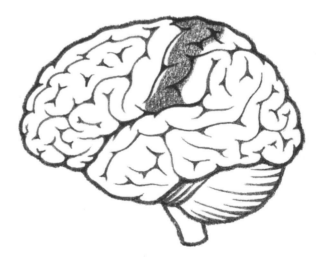

3. _____

4. _____

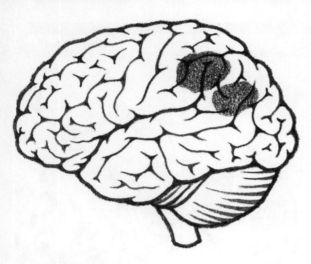

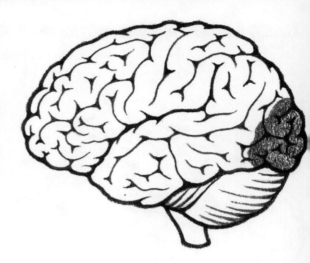

5. _____   6. _____

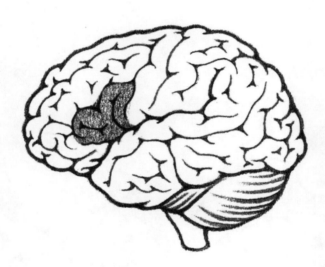

7. _____

Answers to Review Questions

Case Study I

1. a   2. c   3. d   4. a   5. b   6. a   7. d   8. d
9. c

Case Study II

1. c   2. c   3. c   4. a   5. b

Case Study III

1. a   2. a

Case Study IV

1. b   2. b   3. a   4. e   5. b   6. d

Case Study V

1. a   2. a

Case Study VI

1. c   2. b   3. b

Case Study VII

1. a   2. c   3. d

Case Study VIII

1. b   2. a   3. d   4. a   5. b

Case Study IX

1. b   2. a   3. a   4. b

Case Study X

1. b   2. a   3. a   4. b   5. a   6. a

Case Study XI

1. c   2. c   3. a   4. a

Case Study XII

1. a   2. b   3. a   4. b

Case Study XIII

1. b   2. b   3. a

Case Study XIV

1. d   2. c   3. a

Case Study XV

1. a   2. c   3. b

Case Study XVI

1. c   2. c   3. c

Case Study XVII

1. c   2. c   3. c   4. a

Case Study XVIII

1. c   2. a

Case Study XIX

1. c   2. b   3. a

Case Study XX

1. c   2. a   3. b   4. b

Case Study XXI

1. b   2. a   3. b   4. c

Case Study XXII

1. b   2. b   3. a   4. b   5. a   6. a

Case Study XXIII

1. b   2. a

Case Study XXIV

1. e   2. a

Case Study XXV

1. a   2. a

Case Study XXVI

1. b   2. c

Case Study XXVII

1. tactile deficits
2. auditory deficits
3. motor deficits
4. sensory deficits
5. reading, writing, and comprehension deficits
6. visual deficits
7. expressive speech and language deficits

Nerve Supplies to Muscles Important for Swallowing, Speech, and Hearing Functions

The four stages of swallowing are the oral preparatory, oral, pharyngeal, and esophageal. Muscles are used during each stage. The muscles of facial expression, mastication, the soft palate, the tongue, the larynx, and the pharynx are used for swallowing as well as for speech. These muscles are listed along with their nerve supplies.

The muscles used for speech may be divided into muscles that are used for respiration, phonation, resonation, and articulation. In addition, several muscles are used for sound transmission.

Respiration

Muscles used for speech breathing include the major muscle, the diaphragm, which is supplied by the phrenic nerve. The thoracic muscles of respiration (diaphragm, external intercostals, internal intercostals, pectoralis major, pectoralis minor, quadratus lumborum, transverse thoracic, and scalenes) are supplied by peripheral nerves that exit from various levels of the spinal cord. Other abdominal muscles (external oblique, internal oblique, rectus abdominis, transverse abdominis) useful for speech breathing are supplied by the lower intercostals.

Phonation

Muscles used for phonation include the extrinsic and intrinsic muscles of the larynx. All extrinsic muscles (sternohyoid, sternothyroid, thyrohyoid, and omohyoid) inferior to the hyoid bone are supplied by the hypoglossal nerve. The trigeminal, facial, and hypoglossal nerves supply other extrinsic muscles lying superior to the hyoid bone. The digastric and mylohyoid muscles are supplied by the trigeminal nerve. The stylohyoid muscle is supplied by the facial nerve. The geniohyoid muscle is supplied by the hypoglossal nerve. The intrinsic muscles of the larynx (cricothyroid, lateral cricoarytenoid, posterior cricoarytenoid, thyroarytenoid, vocalis, and interarytenoids) are supplied by the vagus nerve.

Resonation

For resonatory function, we use the muscles of the soft palate (levator veli palatine, tensor veli palatine, glossopalatine, pharyngopalatine) and those of the pharynx (superior constrictor, middle constrictor, inferior constrictor, velopharyngeal sphincter, cricopharyngeus, salpingopharyngeus, and stylopharyngeus). The pharyngeal plexus supplies all these muscles except the tensor veli palatine.

Articulation

For speech sound articulation, we use various muscles of facial expression (levator labii superior, levator anguli oris, zygomatic, risorius, depressor anguli oris, depressor anguli superior, mentalis, orbicularis oris, buccinator, and platysma) that are supplied by the facial nerve. We also use muscles of mastication (temporalis, internal pterygoid, external pterygoid, and masseter) that are supplied by the trigeminal nerve. The extrinsic and intrinsic muscles of the tongue are used to articulate specific speech sounds. The three extrinsic muscles (styloglossus, genioglossus, and hyoglossus) are supplied by the hypoglossal nerve. The glossopalatine muscle is supplied by the pharyngeal plexus. The intrinsic muscles (vertical, transverse, inferior longitudinal, and superior longitudinal) are supplied by the hypoglossal nerve.

Sound Transmission

The muscles of the middle ear, which help in sound transmission, are the stapedius and tensor tympani. The stapedius muscle is supplied by the facial nerve, and the tensor tympani muscle is supplied by the trigeminal nerve.

Assessing Adults with Neurogenic Communication Impairment

Once a client with communication and cognitive impairment comes to the clinic, it is important to gather general information, including the client's history and source of referral. After analyzing the symptoms, objective tests are warranted to identify the specific signs of the disease. After these signs are determined, physical and mental processes are examined to formulate the diagnosis and its prognosis. Clinical problem solving is essential at this juncture to arrive at a final diagnosis and start with appropriate intervention.

The purposes of testing clients with neurogenic communication disorders are to diagnose the communication disorder, to arrive at a prognosis by determining the nature and sensitivity of the disorder, and to focus on appropriate treatment paradigms. Before assessing clients with neurogenic disorders, it is essential to know the client's current status, including level of consciousness and severity of language, speech, and cognition impairment. It is also important to understand the family members, their expectations, environmental adjustments, and other related needs. A suitable, justifiable treatment plan can then be developed. Functional communication skills are assessed by asking whether the client communicates within the environment, how communication is accomplished, what is required for communication, etc.

General Assessment for Individuals with Neurogenic Communication Disorders:

- Responsiveness (e.g., levels of arousal, ability to sit, ability to sustain attention, alertness during communication, ability to respond to various visual-auditory-verbal-tactile cues)
- Comprehension (e.g., ability to respond to simple questions, ability to follow simple written directions, ability to follow simple verbal commands)
- Expression (e.g., use of facial expressions, use of pictures or gestures to communicate social greetings, use of a few meaningful phrases)
- Mood (e.g., ability to express emotions, ability to understand others' emotions)

Besides these areas, auditory analysis (e.g., discrimination of word pairs), auditory comprehension (e.g., obtaining meaning from single words), auditory memory (e.g., following two-step directions), graphic abilities, and reading abilities are also analyzed.

Basic neuropsychological assessments in the areas of orientation, attention, visual recognition, visual organization, auditory perception, tactile perception, constructional praxis, visual-verbal memory, executive functions, concept formulation, and personality are done in clients with neurogenic disorders.

The bedside language examination (Alexander & Benson, 1992) is part of the neurological examination and requires an average of 10 to 15 minutes for administration. The test is geared toward understanding the speech/language system so as to arrive at a quick aphasia classification and a possible neuroanatomical localization related to the stroke. Aphasias caused by damage in the anterior language-dominant hemisphere are characterized by nonfluent speech and relatively better language comprehension. Aphasias caused by posterior lesions are apparent by the client's fluent speech but impaired comprehension.

Areas of Assessment in Aphasia

- Listening comprehension
- Reading comprehension
- Speech production
- Linguistic expression
- Cognitive processes

Areas of Assessment in Right Hemisphere Brain Damage Syndrome

- Attention
- Visual and spatial perception
- Recognition and expression of emotion
- Discourse comprehension and production
- Organizational abilities

Areas of Assessment in Traumatic Brain Injury

- Levels of consciousness
- Responsiveness to stimulation
- Orientation
- Cognitive abilities (e.g., memory, judgment, problem-solving abilities)
- Information-processing abilities
- Communication

Areas of Assessment in Dementia

- Orientation
- General knowledge
- Memory
- Communication
- Spatial functions
- Sensation
- Reflexes
- Motor functions

Websites for the Study of Neurology

1. Neuroanatomy
   http://www.neuropat.dote.hu/anatomy.htm
   http://www.meddean.luc.edu/lumen/MedEd/Neuro/Neuro.html
2. Whole brain atlas:
   http://www.med.harvard.edu/AANLIB/home.html
3. Neuropathology atlas
   http://www.neuropat.dote.hu/atlas.html
4. Alzheimer's disease
   http://www.ninds.nih.gov/health_and_medical/disorders/alzheimersdisease_doc.htm
5. Strokes and other neurological disorders
   http://www.stroke.org/
   http://www.mayohealth.org
   http://www.mic.ki.se/Diseases/c10.html
   http://www.ninds.nih.gov
   http://www.alsa.org/
   http://www.parkinson.org/
   www.mdausa.org
   www.aphasia.org
   www.nidcd.nih.gov/health/pubs_vsl/adultaphasia.htm
   www.ninds.nih.gov/health_and_medical/disorders/apraxia.htm
   www.nidcd.nih.gov/health/voice/tbrain.htm
   www.neuro.pmr.vcu.edu
   www.rarediseases.org
   www.williams-syndrome.org
   www.rettsyndrome.org
   www.nofas.org
6. Motor speech disorders
   http://www.ticeinfo.com/speech/index.html
   www.apraxia.org
   www.apraxia-kids.org
   www.cerebralpalsy.org

Appendix 4

Figures of the Brain

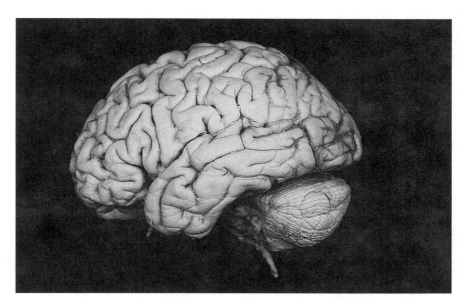

Figure 4-1   Lateral view of the brain. (From Cramer GD, Darby SA: *Basic and clinical anatomy of the spine, spinal cord, and ANS,* St Louis, 1995, Mosby.)

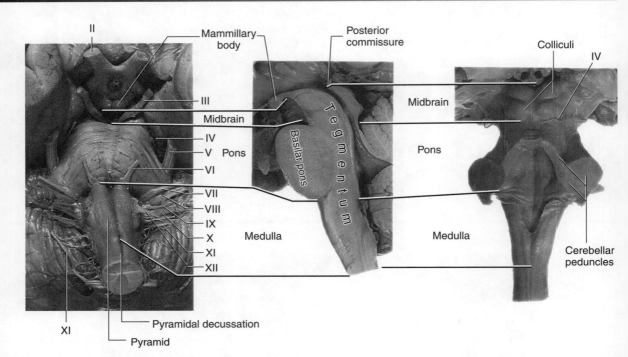

Figure 4-2   Brainstem and origin of cranial nerves. (From Haines DE: *Fundamental neuroscience,* ed 2, Philadelphia, 2002, Churchill Livingstone.)

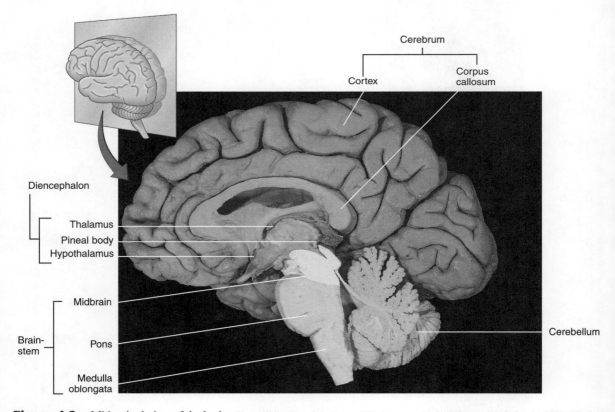

Figure 4-3   Midsagittal view of the brain. (From Thibodeau GA, Patton KT: *Anatomy & physiology,* ed 5, St Louis, 2003, Mosby.)

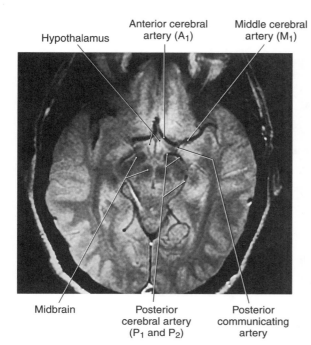

Hypothalamus

Anterior cerebral artery (A₁)

Middle cerebral artery (M₁)

Midbrain

Posterior cerebral artery (P₁ and P₂)

Posterior communicating artery

Figure 4-4 Axial magnetic resonance image showing the circle of Willis. (From Haines DE: *Fundamental neuroscience,* ed 2, Philadelphia, 2002, Churchill Livingstone.)

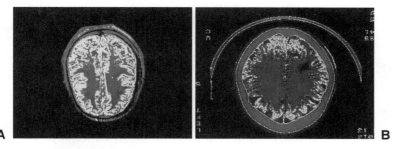

A   B

Figure 4-5 **A,** MRI and **B,** CT scan of the brain. (**A,** Courtesy CNRI/SPL/Photo Researchers; **B,** Courtesy Custom Medical Stock Photo.)

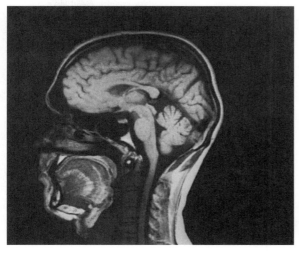

Figure 4-6 MRI of midsagittal view of the brain. (Courtesy Philips Medical Sytems.)

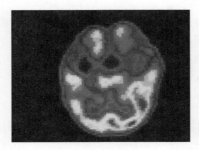

Figure 4-7   PET image of the brain. (Courtesy Dr. Marty Buchsbaum/Peter Arnold, Inc.)

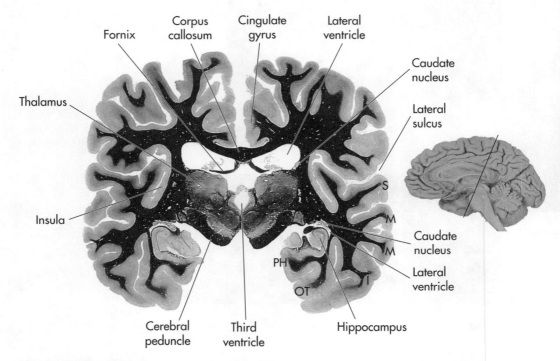

Figure 4-8   Subcortical structures: basal ganglia and thalamus. (From Nolte J: *The human brain: an introduction to its functional anatomy,* ed 5, St Louis, 2002, Mosby.)

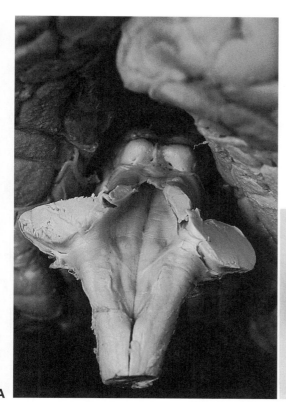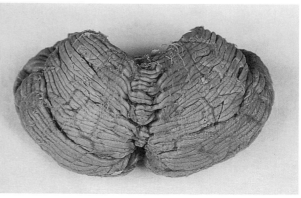

Figure 4-9   Subcortical structures. **A,** Brainstem. **B,** Cerebellum. (From Cramer GD, Darby SA: *Basic and clinical anatomy of the spine, spinal cord, and ANS,* St Louis, 1995, Mosby.)

Two Self-Examinations with Answers

SELF-EXAMINATION I

I. True or False

1. The nervous system is divided into central and peripheral nervous systems.
2. The central nervous system consists of the brain and spinal nerves.
3. Multipolar neurons have a single axon that extends from a small area of the cell body called the axon hillock.
4. The action potential jumps from the sodium channels at one node of Ranvier to the other. This is called saltatory conduction.
5. Microglial cells proliferate at the site of a brain/spinal cord injury in a process called phagocytosis.
6. Astereognosis is the inability to recognize objects by touch.
7. The autonomic nervous system does not include components of the central nervous system.
8. Bradykinesia is seen in Huntington's chorea.
9. The brainstem is situated between the diencephalon and spinal cord.
10. Epilepsy is a peripheral nervous system disorder.
11. Gliosis results from inflammation of the central nervous system.
12. Bipolar neurons are most often motor neurons.
13. The awareness of the body's movement, balance, and position is called proprioception.
14. Multipolar neurons have multiple dendrites and one axon.
15. Basal ganglia is an important component of extrapyramidal system.
16. Temporal summation is the additive summation caused by repeated excitation of a cell membrane.
17. The axon potential is the transient hyperpolarization of the axonal membrane.
18. Schwann cells create myelin sheaths for the central nervous system.
19. Two major arteries that supply blood to the brain are vertebral and external carotid arteries.
20. The space between the arachnoid membrane and pia mater is called the subdural space.

II. Pick the Unrelated Structure

1. dendrite	axon	synapse	tract
2. corpus callosum	arcuate fasciculus	corticobulbar fibers	
3. cortex	pons	midbrain	medulla oblongata
4. thalamus	epithalamus	hypothalamus	substantia nigra
5. astrocytes	oligodendroglia	Schwann cells	microglial cells
6. CT	MRI	x-rays	PET
7. caudate nucleus	putamen	globus pallidus	red nucleus
8. cerebellum	midbrain	pons	medulla oblongata
9. aphasia	apraxia	agnosia	asynergia
10. axon	synapse	bouton	neurotransmitter
11. atrophy	flaccidity	hypertonicity	fasciculations
12. frontal	temporal	parietal	limbic
13. chorea	ballismus	tremor	flaccidity
14. anterior cerebral artery	posterior cerebral artery	anterior communicating artery	middle cerebral artery
15. reticular formation	cranial nerve nuclei	fornix	motor pathways

III. Fill in the Blanks

Expand the abbreviations listed below.

1. CT _____

2. MRI _____

3. CVA _____

4. CSF _____

5. EEG _____

6. EMG _____

7. ENG _____

8. fMRI _____

9. PCA _____

10. PET _____

11. TIA _____

12. LMN _____

13. UMN _____

14. MCA _____

15. ACA _____

IV. Matching

Match the clinical findings with the clinical impressions.

Clinical Findings

1. Inability to comprehend simple commands; inability to name common objects; fluent speech filled with jargon
2. Presence of Babinski's reflex and grasp reflex
3. Occlusive infarct in the posterior branch of the left middle cerebral artery
4. Hyperresponsiveness and impulsivity; perseveration; difficulty with abstract reasoning; impaired self-monitoring; difficulty focusing and sustaining attention
5. Damage in the basal ganglia and extrapyramidal system

Clinical Impressions

hypokinetic dysarthria

traumatic brain injury

Wernicke's aphasia

contralateral corticospinal tract damage

infarction in the left temporoparietal region

V. Multiple Choice

1. Persistent vegetative state is characterized by lack of localizing motor responses, lack of cognition, and inability to follow verbal commands. This is caused by scattered lesions in the _____
   a. central nervous system
   b. peripheral nervous system
   c. autonomic nervous system

2. Locked-in syndrome results from damage in the ventral _____ . No movements are seen except eye blinking and vertical eye movements. The person is mute but conscious.
   a. midbrain
   b. pons
   c. medulla oblongata

3. Signs of increased _____ are papilledema, hypertension, bradycardia, and abducens nerve palsy. Symptoms are headache, nausea and vomiting, diplopia, and decreased levels of consciousness.
   a. intracranial pressure
   b. arterial pressure
   c. venous pressure

4. Criteria for brain death include _____ .
   a. coma or unresponsiveness
   b. absence of auditory evoked potentials
   c. apnea
   d. absence of brainstem reflexes
   e. none of the above
   f. all of the above

5. _____ is a disoriented state often associated with illusions, hallucinations, or incoherent speech.
   a. Agnosia
   b. Amnesia
   c. Delirium
   d. None of the above

6. Disorientation is usually seen in patients with _____ .
   a. dementia
   b. visual disorders
   c. motor disorders
   d. sensory disorders

7. _____ is the unconscious fabrication of events in response to questions about events; it is seen in organic syndromes.
   a. Intrusion
   b. Perseveration
   c. Confabulation

8. _____ amnesia is an impaired ability to learn new material or to form new memories.
   a. Anterograde
   b. Retrograde
   c. Global
   d. Transient

9. _____ amnesia is an impaired ability to recall information that had been known before the onset of illness.
   a. Retrograde
   b. Anterograde
   c. Global
   d. Transient

10. _____ is the repetition of the same response to different questions; it is usually seen in organic mental disorders.
    a. Pallilalia
    b. Perseveration
    c. Paraphasia

11. Functions of glial cells include all of the following except _____ .
    a. structural support
    b. metabolic support
    c. creation of myelin
    d. phagocytosis
    e. conduction of nerve impulses

12. Spinal arteries originate from the _____ artery.
    a. internal carotid
    b. external carotid
    c. vertebral

13. The anteroinferior cerebellar artery emerges from the _____ artery.
    a. vertebral
    b. basilar
    c. internal carotid

VI. Matching

Match the cerebral disorders with the location of their lesions in the dominant hemisphere.

1. Broca's aphasia
2. Wernicke's aphasia
3. Conduction aphasia
4. Transcortical motor aphasia
5. Transcortical sensory aphasia
6. Global aphasia
7. Dyslexia with agraphia

a. Angular gyrus and supramarginal gyrus
b. Frontotemporoparietal areas
c. Inferior to Wernicke's area
d. Auditory association areas
e. Arcuate fasciculus
f. Superior/anterior to the Broca's area
g. Inferior frontal gyrus

VII. Fill in the Blanks

Type of agnosia	Symptoms	Sites of lesion
1. _____	Inability to recognize speech or sound stimuli	Temporoparietal lobes
2. _____	Inability to recognize objects, colors, letters, faces, and places	Parieto-occipital lobes, corpus callosum
3. _____	Inability to recognize objects via touch	Temporoparietal lobes

VIII. Fill in the Blanks

Apraxia is characterized by an inability to carry out a complex movement in the presence of an intact comprehension, motor system, and sensory system.

Type of Apraxia	Symptoms	Sites of Lesion
1. _____	Inability to perform a motor act on command	Parietal lobe, corpus callosum
2. _____	Inability to perform fine motor acts	Frontal lobe
3. _____	Inability to construct a design	Parietal lobe
4. _____	Inability to perform an act based on a sequence of ideas	Parietal lobe
5. _____	Inability to dress	Parietal lobe

IX. Fill in the Blanks

Provide appropriate terms for these descriptions.

1. Inability to perform rapid alternating movements: _____

2. Bundles of nerve fibers that connect symmetrical structures on either side of the central nervous system: _____

3. Involuntary, jerky movements on one side of the body: _____

4. The process of action potential propagation along the length of a myelinated axon where the action potential jumps from one node of Ranvier to the next: _____

5. Brief period after a single action potential: _____

6. Most common type of neuron in the central nervous system: _____

7. Primary function of microglia: _____

8. Arteries that do not directly provide blood to the brain: _____

9. Artery that supplies blood to the inner ear: _____

10. Artery that supplies blood to the temporal lobe of the brain: _____

11. Artery that supplies the corpus striatum: _____

12. Location of lateral ventricles: _____

13. Cerebrospinal fluid is created by this structure: _____

14. Location of alpha and gamma motor neurons: _____

15. A diffuse collection of nuclei in the brainstem that receives various types of sensory input: _____

16. Segment of the brainstem located between the midbrain and the medulla: _____

17. Space created by the juncture of the cerebellum, pons, and medulla: _____

18. Cranial nerves located in the cerebellopontine angle: _____

19. Brodmann's areas 41 and 42: _____

20. Fissure separating the temporal lobe from the parietal and frontal lobes of the cerebrum: _____

21. Gyrus situated dorsal to the corpus callosum: _____

22. Fissure dividing the right and left hemispheres: _____

23. Involuntary patterned motor activity mediated by the spinal cord: _____

24. Organization of frequency-specific placement within the auditory system: _____

25. Region of the cortex concerned with vestibular functions: _____

26. Thalamic nucleus responsible for the visual system: _____

27. System controlling emotions and visceral responses: _____

28. Congenital cleft of the spinal column: _____

29. Sudden paralysis of facial muscles: _____

30. Small brain resulting from early fusion of cranial bones: _____

31. Enlargement of ventricles of the brain because of increased amounts of cerebrospinal fluid:

_____

Answers

I. True or False

1. True	5. True	9. True	13. True	17. False
2. False	6. True	10. False	14. True	18. False
3. True	7. False	11. True	15. True	19. False
4. True	8. False	12. False	16. True	20. False

II. Pick the Unrelated Structure

1. tract
2. corticobulbar fibers
3. cortex
4. substantia nigra
5. Schwann cells
6. PET
7. red nucleus
8. cerebellum
9. asynergia
10. neurotransmitter
11. hypertonicity
12. limbic
13. flaccidity
14. anterior communicating artery
15. fornix

III. Fill in the Blanks

1. computed tomography

2. magnetic resonance imaging

3. cerebrovascular accident

4. cerebrospinal fluid

5. electroencephalography

6. electromyography

7. electronystagmography

8. functional magnetic resonance imaging

9. posterior cerebral artery

10. positron-emission tomography

11. transient ischemic attack

12. lower motor neuron

13. upper motor neuron

14. middle cerebral artery

15. anterior cerebral artery

IV. Matching

1. Wernicke's aphasia
2. contralateral corticospinal tract damage
3. infarction in the left temporoparietal region
4. traumatic brain injury
5. hypokinetic dysarthria

V. Multiple Choice

1. a	3. a	5. c	7. c	9. a	11. e	13. b
2. b	4. f	6. a	8. a	10. b	12. c	

VI. Matching

1. g	2. d	3. e	4. f	5. c	6. b	7. a

VII. Fill in the Blanks

1. Auditory

2. Visual

3. Tactile

VIII. Fill in the Blanks

1. Ideomotor

2. Motor

3. Constructional

4. Ideational

5. Dressing

IX. Fill in the Blanks

1. dysdiadochokinesia

2. corpus callosum

3. hemiballismus

4. saltatory conduction

5. refractory period

6. multipolar neuron

7. phagocytosis

8. posterior and anterior communicating arteries

9. labyrinthine artery

10. middle cerebral artery

11. striate arteries

12. cerebral hemispheres

13. choroid plexus

14. anterior horn of gray matter in the spinal cord

15. reticular formation

16. pons

17. cerebellopontine angle

18. VII and VIII

19. primary auditory areas

20. lateral fissure

21. cingulate gyrus

22. median longitudinal fissure

23. reflex

24. tonotopic organization

25. postcentral gyrus

26. lateral geniculate body

27. limbic system

28. spina bifida

29. facial palsy

30. microcephaly

31. hydrocephalus

SELF-EXAMINATION II
(BASED ON NEUROPATHOLOGY)

1. Trigeminal neuralgia is often caused by _____ .
   a. cross-compression of the trigeminal nerve by arteries
   b. vascular malformations
   c. intrinsic lesions of the brainstem
   d. all of the above
   e. none of the above

2. Temporomandibular joint dysfunction results from _____ .
   a. pain in the jaw or temple
   b. abnormal activities of the tongue
   c. abnormal facial height and width

3. Consciousness is preserved in _____ epilepsy.
   a. simple partial
   b. complex partial
   c. partial seizures with secondary generalization

4. _____ is used to identify pathological changes in patients with intractable focal seizures.
   a. EEG
   b. MRI
   c. CT scan

5. Xth cranial nerve damage leads to paralysis of _____ .
   a. soft palate
   b. pharynx and larynx
   c. tongue
   d. All of the above
   e. All but c

6. Patients with _____ lesions appear to be clumsy, weak, and uncoordinated.
   a. cerebral
   b. basal ganglia
   c. cerebellar

7. _____ is a language dysfunction characterized by comprehension and expression deficits.
   a. Dysarthria
   b. Dysphasia
   c. Dyspraxia

8. A score of 24 to 27 on Mini Mental State Examination indicates _____ dementia.
   a. early
   b. moderate
   c. advanced

9. A defect in the temporal half of one field and the nasal half of another is called _____

   _____ .

   a. altitudinal defect
   b. central scotoma
   c. homonymous hemianopia

10. _____ refers to weakness or incomplete paresis.

    a. Monoplegia
    b. Paralysis
    c. Paresis

11. _____ is a movement disorder characterized by reduced movements.

    a. Bradykinesia
    b. Paraplegia
    c. Tachycardia

12. Eye signs seen in cerebellar diseases include _____ .

    a. abnormal gaze-evoked nystagmus
    b. ocular dysmetria
    c. down-beat nystagmus
    d. all of the above

13. The locked-in syndrome is characterized by _____ .

    a. damage to the corticospinal and corticobulbar tracts
    b. tetraplegia
    c. hypoglycemia
    d. a and b

14. Loss of taste in the anterior two thirds of the tongue, hyperacusis, and loss of lacrimation

    are found in _____ .

    a. upper motor neuron facial weakness
    b. lower motor neuron facial weakness
    c. Ramsay-Hunt syndrome

15. _____ is an involuntary semi-repetitive contraction of muscles around

    the mouth. Involuntary tongue, lip, and jaw movements are also seen.

    a. Myotonia
    b. Hemifacial spasm
    c. Orofacial dyskinesia

16. _____ is a sense of rotation of the individual or the environment.

    a. Fasciculation
    b. Vertigo
    c. Tinnitus

17. _____ produces paroxysmal vertigo, tinnitus, and sensorineural hearing loss.
    a. Seventh cranial nerve palsy
    b. Meniere's disease
    c. Herpes zoster oticus disease

18. _____ degeneration is commonly seen in alcoholic patients and usually affects gait.
    a. Cortical
    b. Cerebellar
    c. Basal ganglia

19. Macroscopically, cortical and subcortical white matter volume is reduced in _____ _____ .
    a. CVA
    b. pontine degeneration
    c. Alzheimer's disease

20. Symptoms of Alzheimer's disease include _____ .
    a. memory loss
    b. depression and personality changes
    c. linguistic disturbances
    d. all of the above

21. To diagnose Lewy body dementia, _____ should be considered.
    a. fluctuating cognitive impairments
    b. extrapyramidal features
    c. transient clouding or loss of consciousness
    d. visual-auditory hallucinations
    e. all of the above but c
    f. all of the above

22. Pick's disease is characterized by _____ .
    a. progressive dementia
    b. reversible dementia
    c. metabolic dementia

23. Nonfluent speech with relatively preserved comprehension is a characteristic of _____ aphasia.
    a. Broca's
    b. Wernicke's
    c. transcortical sensory

24. _____ aphasia(s) is(are) usually characterized by paraphasic errors.
    a. Conduction
    b. Wernicke's
    c. Global
    d. All of the above
    e. None of the above

25. Speech is relatively fluent in _____ aphasia.
    a. Broca's
    b. Wernicke's
    c. transcortical sensory
    d. b and c
    e. none of the above

26. Individuals with Broca's aphasia demonstrate _____ .
    a. dysarthric speech
    b. agnosia
    c. naming deficits
    d. nonfluent speech
    e. all of the above but b
    f. all of the above

27. Repetition is well-preserved in _____ aphasia.
    a. conduction
    b. Broca's
    c. Wernicke's
    d. transcortical

28. In conduction aphasia the site of lesion is in the _____ .
    a. inferior temporal lobe
    b. arcuate fasciculus
    c. middle frontal lobe

29. In Wernicke's aphasia the lesion is located in the _____ .
    a. inferior temporal region of the dominant hemisphere
    b. anterior temporal region of the nondominant hemisphere
    c. posterior temporal region of the dominant hemisphere

30. _____ aphasia is seen as an end result in the recovery of a number of aphasic syndromes.
    a. Sensory
    b. Anomic
    c. Motor

31. Ideational apraxia, which refers to an inability to carry out a sequential motor task, results from a lesion in the _____ lobe.
    a. frontal
    b. temporal
    c. limbic
    d. parietal

32. Ideomotor apraxia may occur with lesions in the _____.
    a. arcuate fasciculus
    b. superior occipital area
    c. premotor cortex
    d. all of the above except b
    e. all of the above

33. _____ with or without agraphia is caused by lesions in the angular gyrus, corpus callosum, and occipital lobe.
    a. Amnesia
    b. Alexia
    c. Agnosia

34. In _____ apraxia the patient is unable to carry out motor commands, although the patient understands them.
    a. verbal
    b. ideomotor
    c. ideational

35. _____ is a disorder of recognition of objects in the absence of loss in any sensory modality.
    a. Aphasia
    b. Agnosia
    c. Apraxia

36. Focal syndromes pertaining to the frontal lobe include _____ .
    a. disinhibition
    b. poor cognition
    c. release of primitive reflexes
    d. all of the above

37. Temporal lobe damage leads to _____ problems.
    a. emotional
    b. memory
    c. a and b
    d. none of the above

38. Right-left disorientation, dyscalculia, dysgraphia, and finger agnosia are characteristics of _____ .
    a. occipital lobe syndrome
    b. Gerstmann's syndrome
    c. Kluver-Bucy syndrome

39. Visual hallucinations are caused by lesions in the _____ lobe.
    a. limbic
    b. parietal
    c. temporal
    d. none of the above

40. _____ is defined as the death of brain tissue as a result of vascular occlusion.
    a. Cerebral infarction
    b. Cerebral hemorrhage
    c. Subarachnoid hemorrhage

41. Cerebral infarction in the internal carotid artery leads to _____ .
    a. dysphasia
    b. blindness
    c. motor disturbances
    d. all of the above

42. Disturbances in the anterior cerebral artery lead to _____ .
    a. sensory loss
    b. apraxia
    c. hemiplegia
    d. transcortical motor aphasia
    e. all of the above

43. Occlusions in the middle cerebral artery result in _____ .
    a. motor and sensory deficits.
    b. homonymous hemianopsia
    c. global aphasia
    d. transcortical motor aphasia
    e. all of the above but d

44. Signs of cerebellar infarction include _____ .
    a. aphasia
    b. sensory deficit
    c. headache and dizziness
    d. gaze paresis and facial paresis
    e. c and d
    f. none of the above

45. Basilar artery occlusions cause _____ .
    a. hydrocephalus
    b. tetraparesis
    c. midbrain damage
    d. altered state of consciousness
    e. all of the above but a
    f. all of the above

46. Brain imaging in Alzheimer's disease shows _____ .
    a. ventricular dilation
    b. cortical atrophy
    c. herniation of the cerebellum
    d. a and b

47. _____ atrophy causes alexia, agraphia, anomia, visual agnosia, and sensory aphasia.
    a. Parieto-occipital
    b. Parietal
    c. Temporal
    d. Frontal

48. Frontal lobe dementia is characterized by changes in _____ .
    a. behavior
    b. language functions
    c. release of extrapyramidal signs
    d. all of the above

49. Presenting symptoms of _____ hematoma include headache, seizures, and decline in intellectual functioning.
    a. subdural
    b. epidural
    c. extradural

50. _____ disease results in bradykinesia, resting tremor, cogwheel rigidity, pill-rolling tremor, and festinating gait.
    a. Parkinson's
    b. Blood vessel
    c. Pick's

51. Tremor is related to rhythmic neuronal discharge in the _____ .
    a. corpus callosum
    b. thalamus
    c. brainstem

52. Progressive supranuclear palsy is caused by lesions in the _____ .
    a. subthalamic nuclei
    b. brainstem
    c. corpus striatum
    d. all of the above

53. Clinical manifestations of cerebral tumors include _____ .
    a. headache
    b. seizures and altered mental status
    c. memory deficits
    d. all of the above

54. Focal symptoms of _____ lobe lesions include altered mood and behavior.
    a. parietal
    b. frontal
    c. occipital

55. Focal symptoms of _____ lobe lesions include sensory deficits, apraxia, and visual deficits.
    a. parietal
    b. frontal
    c. temporal

56. _____ is a sign of increased intracranial pressure resulting from the presence of tumors.
    a. Fourth cranial nerve palsy
    b. Third cranial nerve palsy
    c. Papilledema

57. Symptoms of a cortical lesion include _____ .
    a. aphasia
    b. apraxia
    c. homonymous hemianopia
    d. a and b
    e. all of the above

58. Symptoms of a subcortical lesion include _____ .
    a. involuntary movements
    b. contralateral hemiplegia
    c. a and b
    d. none of the above

59. Temporal lobe deficits result in _____ .
    a. limited concentration
    b. uninhibited social behavior
    c. painful sensations
    d. receptive aphasias

60. Incoordination of motor movements is associated with _____ lesions.
    a. cerebellar
    b. cerebral
    c. brainstem

61. Inattention, spatial and temporal disorientation, and prosapagnosia are symptoms of lesions in the _____ .
    a. nondominant hemisphere
    b. dominant hemisphere
    c. internal capsule
    d. brainstem

62. Bilateral loss of pain and temperature sensation implies a lesion in the _____ .
    a. white matter of the spinal cord
    b. gray matter of the spinal cord
    c. brainstem

63. _____ is associated with a lesion in the optic tract fibers.
    a. Bitemporal hemianopia
    b. Homonymous hemianopia
    c. Visual agnosia

64. Visual agnosia is associated with lesions in the _____ .
    a. visual cortex
    b. optic chiasm
    c. optic tract

65. Hypotonia, hyporeflexia, and atrophy are related to lesions in the _____ .
    a. upper motor neurons
    b. lower motor neurons
    c. spinal cord

66. Cranial nerve deficits, vertigo, nystagmus, altered consciousness, and ocular problems are associated with damage in the _____ .
    a. basal ganglia
    b. spinal cord
    c. brainstem

67. Increased involuntary movements, abnormal posture, and bradykinesia are associated with lesions in the _____ .
    a. brainstem
    b. basal ganglia
    c. thalamus

68. Impaired tactile discrimination and constructional apraxia are associated with _____ lobe lesions.
    a. temporal
    b. parietal
    c. frontal
    d. none of the above

69. Early hemorrhagic transformations in the brain can easily be detected with the help of _____ .
    a. CT
    b. MRI
    c. EEG

70. Hematoma in the _____ results in contralateral sensorimotor deficits and ocular problems.
    a. spinal cord
    b. putamen
    c. thalamus
    d. b and c

71. Vomiting, headache, vertigo, ataxia, altered consciousness, and dysarthria are symptoms of _____ hematoma.
    a. occipital lobe
    b. cerebellar
    c. frontal lobe

72. Vascular malformations in the brain may be viewed by _____ .
    a. EMG
    b. angiography
    c. EEG

73. Subarachnoid hemorrhage is usually caused by the rupture of _____ .
    a. veins
    b. tumors
    c. aneurysms

74. Glioblastoma multiforme is a tumor that arises from _____ .
    a. oligodendrocytes
    b. microglia
    c. astrocytes

75. General symptoms of cerebral tumors include _____ .
    a. seizures
    b. nausea
    c. vomiting
    d. headache
    e. all of the above

76. The hallmark sign of multiple sclerosis is _____ .
    a. multiple tumors in the spinal cord
    b. CNS demyelination
    c. Wallerian degeneration

77. Early symptoms of multiple sclerosis include _____ .
    a. diplopia
    b. sensory and motor disturbances
    c. balance disorders
    d. aphasia
    e. all of the above but d

78. Symptoms of bacterial meningitis include _____ .
    a. headache
    b. malaise
    c. photophobia
    d. all of the above

79. Signs and symptoms of _____ include the insidious onset of altered cognitive behaviors, personality changes, and motor incoordination.
    a. spinal cord injury
    b. meningitis
    c. AIDS dementia complex

80. Amyotrophic lateral sclerosis is a type of _____ disturbance.
    a. sensory
    b. motor neuron
    c. autonomic nervous system

81. Upper motor neuron signs include _____ .
    a. hypertonia
    b. hyperreflexia
    c. spasticity
    d. fasciculation
    e. all of the above but d

82. Progressive bulbar palsy is a condition characterized by _____ .
    a. dysphagia
    b. dysarthria
    c. emotional lability
    d. all of the above

83. EMG criteria for diagnosing motor neuron disease include _____ .
    a. reduction of action potentials
    b. abnormal sensory conduction
    c. fasciculations and fibrillations
    d. all of the above
    e. all of the above but b

84. Muscular weakness exaggerates with fatigue in _____ .
    a. poliomyelitis
    b. Parkinson's disease
    c. myasthenia gravis

85. Duchenne muscular dystrophy is not characterized by _____ .
    a. gait disturbances
    b. cognitive deficiencies
    c. dysarthria
    d. apraxia

Answers:

1. d	12. d	23. a	34. b	45. e	56. c	67. b	78. d
2. a	13. d	24. d	35. b	46. d	57. e	68. b	79. c
3. a	14. b	25. d	36. d	47. a	58. c	69. b	80. b
4. b	15. c	26. e	37. c	48. d	59. d	70. d	81. e
5. e	16. b	27. d	38. b	49. a	60. a	71. b	82. d
6. c	17. b	28 b	39. d	50. a	61. a	72. b	83. e
7. b	18. b	29. c	40. a	51. b	62. b	73. c	84. c
8. a	19. c	30. b	41. d	52. d	63. b	74. c	85. d
9. c	20. d	31. a	42. e	53. d	64. a	75. e	
10. c	21. e	32. d	43. e	54. b	65. b	76. b	
11. a	22. a	33. b	44. e	55. a	66. c	77. e	

Glossary

Action potential: Change in electrical potential from a negative to a more positive value.

Afferent: Sensory nerves that carry information from the periphery to the central nervous system.

Agraphia: Impaired writing resulting from frontal and parietal lobe damage.

Alexia without agraphia: Inability to read but retention of writing ability; caused by disconnection of visual cortex from Wernicke's area.

Alzheimer's disease: Progressive degenerative disease of the brain characterized by cognitive and linguistic disturbances.

Amygdaloid nucleus: Structure attached to the caudal end of caudate nucleus; involved with emotional behaviors.

Amyotrophic lateral sclerosis: Degenerative condition of the nervous system characterized by lower and upper motor neurons.

Anesthesia: Complete loss of sensation.

Aneurysm: Balloon-like bulges in an artery caused by weakness in the arterial wall.

Angular gyrus: Structure located near the end of the superior temporal sulcus important for the integration of auditory, visual, and somatosensory information.

Anterior horn cells: Spinal motor neurons located in the anterolateral part of the spinal cord.

Arachnoid villi: Sites at which resorption of cerebrospinal fluid takes place.

Arcuate fasciculus: Fibers that connect the frontal and occipital lobes and are important for language and memory.

Arteriovenous malformations: Collection of weak veins and arteries that are susceptible to rupture.

Association cortex: Areas of the cerebral cortex that do not receive direct input and are involved in higher level processing of sensory and motor information.

Association fibers: Fibers confined within each hemisphere that connect cortical areas.

Ataxia: Loss of motor coordination resulting from a lesion in the cerebellum.

Atrophy: Wasting away of muscles.

Autonomic nervous system: Also called involuntary nervous system; innervates visceral organs and glands.

Axon: Long conducting process of the neuron.

Basal ganglia: Gray matter masses located deep inside the brain; responsible for muscle movements and tone.

Basilar artery: Formed by connections of two vertebral arteries.

Bell's palsy: Ipsilateral paralysis of lower facial muscles caused by lower motor neuron lesion involving the facial nerve nucleus.

Blood-brain barrier: Barrier lining the blood vessels of the brain formed by astrocytes.

Brain abscess: Cavity in the brain caused by various infections.

Brainstem: Stalklike structure that connects the brain to the spinal cord.

Broca's area: Area of the cortex in the inferior convolution of the frontal lobe important for expressive speech.

Central fissure: Also known as the fissure of Rolando; divides the brain into anterior and posterior halves.

Central nervous system: Consists of the brain and spinal cord. This system serves for cognition, language, perception, sensorimotor integration, regulation of motor movements, reflexes, and vital body functions, such as respiration, heartbeat, etc.

Cerebellum: Structure that lies posterior to the brainstem and inferior to the cerebrum; helps in coordination of movements of muscles and equilibrium.

Cerebral aqueduct: Connection between the third and fourth ventricles.

Cerebral palsy: Nonprogressive motor disorder caused by damage to cortical and subcortical structures.

Cerebrovascular accident: Sensorimotor disturbances caused by lack of blood supply to the brain.

Cerebrum: Also known as the telencephalon, which is the main portion of the brain occupying upper part of the cranium. It consists of two cerebral hemispheres (right and left) connected by the corpus callosum. It serves cognitive, linguistic, sensorimotor, and perceptual functions.

Cerebrospinal fluid: Clear, colorless fluid that fills the ventricles and protects the central nervous system from shocks or damage.

Chorea: Disorder, characterized by quick dancelike movements, that results from damage in the subthalamic nuclei.

Choroid plexus: Network of capillaries situated in each ventricle for producing cerebrospinal fluid.

Circle of Willis: Vascular arrangement on the base of the brain formed by vertebral and internal carotid arteries.

Commissural fibers: Fibers that cross between the hemispheres of the brain (e.g., corpus callosum).

Contralateral organization: Left cortex controls sensory and motor functions of the right half of the body and vice versa.

Corona radiata: Fanlike structure of sensorimotor fibers that extends from the internal capsule to the cerebral cortex.

Corpus callosum: Bundle of commissural fibers that connect two cerebral hemispheres.

Cortex: Outer layer of the cerebral hemispheres.

Corticobulbar tract: Motor tract traveling from the cortex to the brainstem.

Corticospinal tract: Motor tract traveling from the cortex to the spinal cord.

Cranial vault: Space inside the skull that houses the brain.

Decussation: Crossing of nerve fibers in the midline.

Dementia: Impairment of intellect and cognition secondary to several reversible and irreversible nervous system diseases.

Demyelination: Process of breaking down the myelin sheaths that cover the axons within neurons.

Dendrites: Processes of a neuron that receives many synapses.

Diencephalon: Portion of the brain that includes subcortical masses such as the thalamus and hypothalamus.

Dorsal cochlear nucleus: Structure located in the medulla that is important for audition.

Dorsal columns: Structures located in the spinal cord that transmit information about touch sensations.

Dorsal horn: Dorsal part of the central gray matter of the spinal cord.

Dura mater: Connective tissue supporting the brain.

Dysarthria: Speech impairment secondary to damage in the nervous system.

Dyskinesia: Abnormal and involuntary muscle movements that are caused by extrapyramidal lesions.

Dyslexia: Reading impairment.

Dystonia: Spasmodic contraction of muscles.

Efferent: Describes nerves carrying information away from the central nervous system to the periphery.

Epilepsy: Disorder resulting from abnormal electrical activities in the brain; characterized by sensorimotor and cognitive disturbances.

Extrapyramidal system: Motor pathways that control muscle tone and help regulate motor movements.

Falx cerebelli: Continuation of dura mater into the median longitudinal fissure.

Fasciculus: Several parallel-running tracts composed of white matter.

Fibrillation: Contraction of single muscle fibers.

Fissure: Deep sulcus (e.g., median longitudinal fissure).

Focal lesion: Lesion that can be pinpointed.

Foramen magnum: Structure through which the brainstem, nerves, and blood vessels pass; connects the brain and spinal cord.

Fornix: An archlike structure inferior to the corpus callosum, seen on the medial section of the brain. It consists of pathways that mediate connections among the hippocampus, hypothalamus, and septum pellucidum to serve various visceral functions and memory.

Functional plasticity: Ability to reorganize and modify functions as a result of a repair of the cortical circuitry.

Ganglion: Collection of cell bodies of neurons.

Glial cells: Supporting tissue of the brain.

Glioblastoma multiforme: Malignant tumor of glial cells.

Granulovacuolar degeneration: Fluid-filled cavities within nerve cells; typically seen in Alzheimer's disease.

Gray matter: Region of the central nervous system that consists of neuronal cell bodies.

Hematoma: Accumulation of blood from a hemorrhage.

Hemianopia: Blindness in half of the visual field.

Hemiplegia: Paralysis of one side of the body.

Herniation: Displacement of brain tissue.

Heschl's gyrus: Primary auditory area located in the superior gyrus of the temporal lobe.

Hippocampus: Structure found deep in the brain beneath the parahippocampal gyrus; related to formation of short-term memory.

Huntington's chorea: Progressive degenerative disease of the brain caused by extrapyramidal lesions and leading to dementia and chorea.

Hydrocephalus: Disorder caused by obstruction in the flow of cerebrospinal fluid; results in an enlarged head and dilation of ventricles.

Hypoperfusion: Diminished blood supply.

Hypothalamus: Structure located near the thalamus that helps mediate food intake, osmotic balances, and control of autonomic nervous system.

Inferior colliculus: Nuclei in the midbrain responsible for audition.

Insular cortex: Also called the island of Reil; situated in the depth of the lateral fissure.

Internal capsule: Space between the thalamus and basal ganglia through which nerve fibers pass.

Interneuron: Neuron with a short axon.

Lateral fissure: Divides the frontal lobe from the parietal lobe.

Lateral geniculate body: Nucleus in the thalamus that relays visual information to the primary visual cortex.

Lateral spinothalamic tract: Axons from the spinal cord to the thalamus transmitting information regarding pain and temperature.

Lemniscus: Bundle of nerve fibers in the central nervous system.

Limbic lobe: Structure consisting of the hippocampus, parahippocampal gyrus, uncus, subcallosal gyrus, and cingulate gyrus; deals with emotional behaviors.

Localization of symptoms: Clinical symptoms in neurologically damaged patients related to specific regions in the nervous system.

Medial geniculate body: Nucleus in the thalamus constituting the auditory pathway that sends axons to the auditory cortex.

Medulla: Inferiormost structure of the brainstem that regulates respiration, phonation, heartbeat, etc.

Meninges: Membranes between the skull and the brain that act as protective layers.

Midbrain: Superiormost part of the brainstem responsible for motor movements and auditory and visual reflexes; contains nuclei of cranial nerves, substantia nigra, and red nucleus.

Myoclonus: Fine, rapid, irregular contractions of muscles.

Neoplasm: Benign or malignant tumors that destroy surrounding normal tissues.

Neuralgia: Pain caused by the inflammation of nerves.

Neuritic plaques: Areas of nerve cell degeneration.

Neuroanatomy: Subdivision of neurology that studies the anatomy of nervous tissue and the nervous system.

Neurofibrillary tangles: Filamentous bodies in the cell body, dendrites, axon, and synapses; typically seen in Alzheimer's disease.

Neurology: Study of the nervous system, especially its structure, functions, and abnormalities; focuses on the diagnosis and treatment of disorders pertaining to the central and peripheral nervous systems.

Neuromuscular junction: Synapse between a motor neuron and a muscle cell.

Neuropathology: Study of diseases and their effects on the nervous system.

Neurophysiology: Study of the chemical, electrical, and metabolic functions of the nervous system.

Neuroradiology: Study of diagnostic techniques used for various nervous system disorders.

Nucleus: Mass of neurons situated deep in the brain.

Nystagmus: Abnormal movements of eyes caused by balance and equilibrium disorders.

Optic chiasm: Point at which optic fibers cross.

Optic radiation: Visual pathway between the retina of the eye and the cortex.

Parasympathetic nervous system: Parts of the autonomic nervous system that deals with relaxation of sympathetic activation.

Paresthesia: Abnormal sensations in absence of stimuli.

Parkinson's disease: Progressive disease of the brain characterized by resting tremor, bradykinesia, and rigidity.

Pia mater: Very thin layer rich in capillaries that is closely attached to the contours of the brain.

Planum temporale: Area on the left temporal lobe that is important for language functions.

Postcentral gyrus: Primary sensory cortex posterior to the central fissure.

Precentral gyrus: Primary motor cortex anterior to the central fissure.

Projection fibers: Fibers that carry sensory and motor information and connect the cortex with the brainstem and spinal cord.

Pyramidal system: Motor pathways that initiate voluntary movements.

Reflex: Stereotyped and specific response to a specific stimulus without the participation of the cortex.

Reticular formation: Cells on the brainstem structures that control the overall level of consciousness.

Schwann cell: Type of glial cell in the peripheral nervous system that produces myelin.

Seizures: Abnormal patterns of neuronal discharge in the brain.

Sensory memory: Area where traces of stimuli are briefly stored for processing of information.

Spasticity: Characterized by hypertonia and hyperreflexia secondary to upper motor neuron damage.

Spinal cord: Structure belonging to the central nervous system that regulates reflexes.

Substantia nigra: Structure in the midbrain responsible for movement.

Superior colliculus: Nuclei on the tectum of the midbrain responsible for controlling eye movements.

Sympathetic nervous system: Part of the autonomic nervous system that deals with fight, flight, or fear responses.

Synaptic cleft: Gap separating the presynaptic from the postsynaptic membrane.

Synaptic vesicles: Sacs containing neurotransmitters; found in the synaptic knobs of the axons.

Thalamus: Relay station for all sensory information coming from the brain and the body.

Tonotopic organization: Anatomic arrangement in the auditory nerve cells in order of increasing frequency of response.

Tract: Collection of axons that run in parallel.

Transient ischemic attack: Temporary disruption of cerebral circulation that causes sensory, motor, and mental disturbances.

Ventral horn: Ventral part of the gray matter of the spinal cord containing the cell bodies of motor neurons.

Ventricles: Fluid-filled centers of the brain.

Ventrocochlear nucleus: Nucleus in the medulla responsible for audition.

Wernicke-Korsakoff syndrome: Disorder caused by alcohol abuse; characterized by amnesia, psychosis, and language disturbances.

White matter: Bundles of myelinated axons.

Bibliography

Alexander, M.P., & Benson, D.F. (1992). In Joynt, R.J. (Ed.). *Clinical neurology.* Philadelphia: JB Lippincott.

Aronson, A.E. (2000). *Aronson's neurosciences pocket lectures.* San Diego: Singular Publishing.

Barr, M.L., & Kiernan, J.A. (1983). *The human nervous system: an anatomical viewpoint.* (4th ed.). Philadelphia: Harper & Row.

Berkow, R., Beers, M.H., & Fletcher, A.J. (1997). *The Merck manual of medical information.* (Home ed.). Whitehouse Station, NJ: Merck Research Laboratories.

Bhatnagar, S.C., & Andy, O.J. (1995). *Neuroscience for the study of communicative disorders.* Baltimore: Williams & Wilkins.

Boron, W., & Boulpaep, E. (2003). *Medical physiology.* Philadelphia: W.B. Saunders.

Brookshire, R.H. (1997). *Introduction to neurogenic communication disorders.* (5th ed.). St. Louis: Mosby.

Cohen, H. (1999). *Neuroscience for rehabilitation.* (2nd ed.). Philadelphia: Lippincott Williams & Wilkins.

Donaghy, M. (1997). *Neurology.* Oxford: Oxford University Press.

Dworkin, J.P., & Hartman, D.E. (1994). *Cases in neurogenic communication disorders.* (2nd ed.). San Diego: Singular Publishing.

Freed, D.B. (2000). *Motor speech disorders.* San Diego: Singular Thompson Learning.

Gertz, S.D. (1991). *Liebman's neuroanatomy made easy and understandable.* (6th ed.). Frederick, Md.: Aspen.

Haines, D.E. (2002). *Fundamental neuroscience,* (2nd ed.), Philadelphia: Churchill Livingstone.

Haines, D.E. (2000). *Neuroanatomy: an atlas of structures, sections, and systems.* (5th ed.). Philadelphia: Lippincott Williams & Wilkins.

Halpern, H. (2000). *Language and motor speech disorders in adults.* Austin, Tex.: Pro-Ed.

Hiatt, J.L., & Gartner, L.P. (2001). *Textbook of head and neck anatomy.* (3rd ed.). Philadelphia: Lippincott Williams & Wilkins.

Kirshner, H.S. (1995). *Handbook of neurological speech and language disorders.* New York: Marcel Dekker.

Kolb, B., & Whishaw, P. (1990). *Fundamentals of human neuropsychology.* (3rd ed.). New York: W.H. Freeman.

Larson, D.E. (1990). *Mayo Clinic family health book.* New York: William Morrow.

Love, R.J., & Webb, W.G. (2001). *Neurology for the speech-language pathologist.* (4th ed.). Boston: Butterworth-Heinemann.

Nolte J. (2002). *The human brain: an introduction to its functional anatomy* (5th ed.). St. Louis: Mosby.

Oishi, M. (1997). *Handbook of neurology.* New Jersey: World Scientific.

Palmer, J. (1993). *Anatomy for speech and hearing.* (4th ed.). Philadelphia: Lippincott Williams & Wilkins.

Perkin, G.A. (1998). *Mosby's color atlas and text of neurology.* London: Mosby.

Peters, A., Palay, S.L., & Webster, H. (1991). *The fine structures of the nervous system: neurons and their supporting cells.* (3rd ed.). New York: Oxford University Press.

Schmidt, R.F. (1985). *Fundamentals of neurophysiology.* (3rd rev. ed.). New York: Springer-Verlag.

Watson, C. (1977). *Basic human neuroanatomy.* (2nd ed.). Boston: Little, Brown.

Waxman, S.G. (2000). *Correlative neuroanatomy.* New York: Lange Medical Books/McGraw Hill.

Webster, D.B. (1999). *Neuroscience of communication.* (2nd ed.). San Diego: Singular Publishing.

Weiner, W.J., & Goetz, C.G. (1999). *Neurology for the non-neurologist.* Philadelphia: Lippincott Williams & Wilkins.

Index

Page numbers followed by *f* indicate figures;
t, tables; *b,* boxes.